Fit As Fido

Nancy -
Let Onzy be your own
"canine personal trainer"
to show you how to be
fit and fabulous!
Dawn Marcus, MD
www.FitAsFido.com

Wheatie

Toby

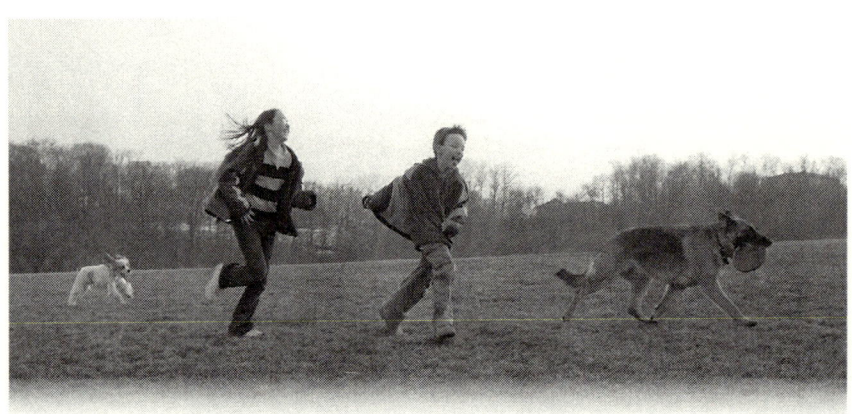

There are so many ways "our" best friends enrich our lives. Not only do dogs provide us with that emotional lift we so desperately need by taking care of our mental health, in *Fit As Fido*, Dr. Marcus provides yet another positive result of human-canine companionship demonstrating how our 4-legged therapists help us to become physically healthy as well.

Shawn Bengston
Professional dog trainer

Fit As Fido

✦

Follow Your Dog to Better Health

Dawn A. Marcus, MD

iUniverse, Inc.
New York Bloomington

Fit As Fido

Follow Your Dog to Better Health

Copyright © 2008 by Dawn A. Marcus, MD

All rights reserved. No part of this book may be used or reproduced by any means, graphic, electronic, or mechanical, including photocopying, recording, taping or by any information storage retrieval system without the written permission of the publisher except in the case of brief quotations embodied in critical articles and reviews.

iUniverse books may be ordered through booksellers or by contacting:

iUniverse
1663 Liberty Drive
Bloomington, IN 47403
www.iuniverse.com
1-800-Authors (1-800-288-4677)

Because of the dynamic nature of the Internet, any Web addresses or links contained in this book may have changed since publication and may no longer be valid. The views expressed in this work are solely those of the author and do not necessarily reflect the views of the publisher, and the publisher hereby disclaims any responsibility for them.

ISBN: 978-0-595-53101-1 (pbk)
ISBN: 978-0-595-63161-2 (ebk)
ISBN: 978-0-595-51844-9 (cloth)

Printed in the United State of America

Library of Congress Control Number: 2008940939

iUniverse rev. date: 01/07/2009

Cover photo courtesy of Donna Hudson
www.fitasfido.com

Acknowledgement

I would like to give a special thanks to those who shared their dogs' photos with me for this book: Joyce Arnowitz, Shawn Bengston, Susan Borzelleca, Donna Hudson, Anne Marie Klipa, Sherry Meininghaus, Julie Milone, Cheryl Noethiger, Susan Showalter, and Jillian Williams.

Note:

This book is not intended to provide individual medical advice. Individuals needing expert assistance should contact their healthcare providers for personalized recommendations.

Foreword

For thousands of years, humans and dogs have had a deep connection—as hunting partners, companions, workmates and playmates. Now science is proving that the relationship between pets and pet parents is even more significant. The simple fact is: you and your pet are good for each other in ways you may have never imagined.

For example, studies show that owning a pet increases your activity level while lowering your blood pressure and cholesterol. And service animals can help people physically and mentally.

As a doctor of medicine and a lover of dogs, Dawn Marcus is the perfect guide to explain how much you and your pet can do for each other.

In addition to being a respected author, Dr. Marcus is a consultant to Del Monte's "Power of Paws" program, which explores how your relationship with your pet can help improve the lives of others. She participates in the "Ask the Experts" page on our website, www.PowerOfPaws.com.

Del Monte is proud to provide the foods that keep your pet happy and fit. Because, as Dr. Marcus shows, the benefits go both ways.

Lisa Henriksen
VP, Innovation & Business Development
Del Monte Pet Products

Preface

"You've got to be kidding!" These were the words of dismay uttered by my husband when my 16-year-old son announced he'd like a puppy for his birthday. During our twenty years of marriage, we'd never had a dog. We'd spent our first 10 years in apartments while we put ourselves through school and began medical practices. We'd briefly entertained getting a dog when the boys were young, but saw how our friends were tied down with their dog responsibilities and unable to enjoy the frequent and extended traveling our family appreciated. The last few years had been monopolized with our sons' school, Boy Scouts, and after-school sports activities. Now that the boys were just a couple of years away from heading off to college, did we really want to saddle ourselves down with a dog?

My husband grew up in apartments in New York City, where dogs were not welcome. I had grown up with dogs—my dad was an avid pheasant and quail hunter, while my artist mother painted portraits of show dogs. When I was born, my parents decided to get an English springer spaniel puppy for my 2-year-old brother. Skipper and I grew up together and he became my constant friend, companion, and confidant for the next 12 years until my dad filled our house with pointers. Like most dogs in my country neighborhood, mine left the house early each morning, spent his days running and hunting in the woods, and then returned home exhausted each evening. His life was quite different from that of the suburban dog who is often adopted as a pampered member of the family rather than a worker.

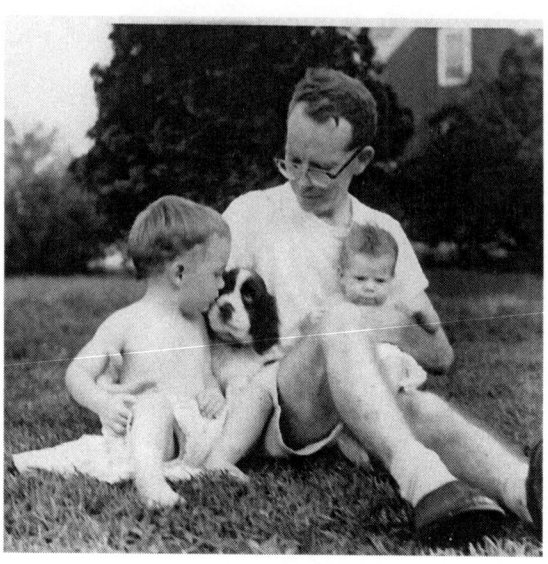

New puppy and baby. I'm the perplexed-looking one on the right.

So after years of having fish, salamanders, and birds in the house, we finally took the plunge and found a perfect little puppy. In the pet world, fish often appear bored, cats aloof, and gerbils busily anxious. But the dog is the pet that has the air of contentment. The dog is at peace with himself and his home. As new owners, we often marveled at how quickly our little pooch adapted to new adventures in the country, city, or suburb.

When we welcomed a soft-coated wheaten terrier pup into our lives, he soon accompanied us on frequent weekend trips to our sons' sporting events, camping, and college tours. Whether finding himself in the North or South, tent or hotel, sun or rain, the little terrier remained satisfied, with a wag in his tail and a bounce in his step. While, we humans grumbled about long drives, uncomfortable temperatures, and unfamiliar surroundings, the little dog enthusiastically embraced each new situation as a novel adventure to enjoy.

As a doctor, I spend most of my days listening to people's problems and helping them to modify their lives to reduce unpleasant physical and emotional symptoms. Although medical school focused on the miracles of modern medications, my practice taught me that a bottle of pills is usually only a small part of each patient's necessary prescription package. In order to truly improve one's health, most patients need changes in their physical activity, eating habits, sleeping patterns, and approaches to stress and social situations. Being in charge of a pet as an adult, I soon discovered that the same lessons I preached to my patients could be mirrored by training practices with my wheaten pup. Like many of my patients, Wheatie could be a star pupil when he ate, slept, and exercised adequately and on schedule—and a terrier terror if I got lazy and allowed him to get into my bad habits. I also discovered my own health improved, once I followed the training regimen my son and I had posted on the refrigerator for Wheatie. Eating, sleeping, and exercising with him helped me develop practical tips on how my patients might better adopt healthy lifestyle habits.

Living with a contented terrier provides a welcome contrast to the high-stress, road-rage, enough-is-never-enough encounters one meets daily at home, work, shopping, or even dining out. There's a lot one can learn from man's best friend about approaching life with a positive attitude and adopting a healthy lifestyle. Your dog can become a terrific role model for better living.

Fortunately, learning from a dog is easy. The Humane Society estimates that about 65 million dogs are owned as pets (www.hsus.org). This means that almost 40 percent of all homes in the United States have a pet dog. If you're looking for a dog, there's great advice about choosing the breed that's best for you from the American Kennel Club (www.akc.org), the Humane Society (www.hsus.org), and the website selectsmart.com. Once you've found a breed that might be right for you, contact experts at your local shelters and breed-specific rescue organizations to get more detailed information to ensure this will be the right fit for you and your family.

This book is designed to help motivate you to learn from your dog to improve your health. Dog owners taking advantage of the possible health benefits of having a canine in their lives can experience improved physical and mental fitness. So welcome instruction from your canine personal trainer—learn to live the dog's life and enjoy better health and happiness.

Dawn A. Marcus, MD

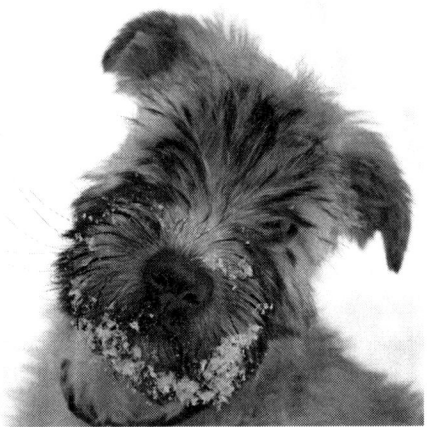

Let Wheatie guide you to a healthier lifestyle.

About the author

Dawn A. Marcus, MD is a board-certified neurologist and professor at the University of Pittsburgh Medical Center. While spending two decades managing patients with chronic pain complaints, she soon learned that treatments required more than simply improving the physical status of damaged joints, muscles, and nerves. These patients really required a holistic approach—treating their diet, sleep patterns, exercise habits, mood, and social concerns. Substantial improvements generally occurred only after patients had received necessary attention to their physical, psychological, social, and family problems.

Dr. Marcus is a nationally and internationally recognized speaker and educator of doctors, nurses, and lay people. Lessons learned through years of successfully treating patients with chronic pain have been condensed into practical, easy-to-read resources for both doctors and patients. She has published over 100 articles in medical journals and is the author of numerous book chapters and six medical books, including *10 Simple Solutions to Migraines, Headache and Chronic Pain Syndromes: The Case-Based Guide to Targeted Assessment and Treatment*, and *Headache Simplified*. She has been the lead investigator for numerous research studies, including studies investigating the benefits of exercise, relaxation therapy, and biofeedback in adults and children. You can find a number of educational materials she has designed for patients on her website: www.dawnmarcusmd.com. Dr. Marcus welcomes feedback from readers visiting her website, where you may post your book reviews and comments.

Dr. Marcus grew up on a beautiful, wooded 40-acre plot in upstate New York, surrounded by enthusiastic and well-trained hunting dogs. After settling with her family in Pittsburgh, a delightful wheaten terrier entered her home, resulting in health benefits for her, her husband, and her teenage boys. The little terrier soon became instructor to the professor, teaching many valuable lessons about healthy living and a positive attitude. Through terrier training, she's more active, happier, and 20 pounds lighter!

Contents

Acknowledgement v

Note: v

Enjoy the Health Benefits of Having a Dog 1

Eat Like a Dog 25

Play Like a Dog 51

Sleep Like a Dog 69

Be Man's Best Friend 85

Teach an Old Dog New Tricks 96

Live a Dog's Life 106

Chapter 1.

Enjoy the Health Benefits of Having a Dog

I'm 40 years old and the mother of three teenagers. Between driving them to soccer, baseball, and band practices and trying to keep the house in some order, there's no time to work out at the gym or cook special health foods. And I have a basement full of the latest fads in at-home exercise equipment. Last year, we inherited my nephew's big retriever and now I spend all day vacuuming up his hair. I'll never get myself in shape. HELP!
Julie N., Pittsburgh, PA

Who doesn't want to lead a healthier life? Television advertisements and Internet pop-ups promise superior health with lots of treatments. Kind of reminds you of the snake venom salesman from the 1800's, peddling his cure-all potion from the back of a rickety wagon. With so many pills, potions, and machines available with the touch of the phone or click of a mouse, your home can become full of an assortment of never-to-be-used wonders.

Take note of how your dog lives his life—how he eats, plays, sleeps, and interacts with others around him. Mirroring simple aspects of your life on the habits of Lucky as your role model will improve both your physical and mental health. This book is designed to teach you how to begin to live a healthier life—following Tracker as your guide. You will learn the dog way to approach many aspects of daily living from how you prepare your foods—to how to schedule enough exercise and sleep—to how you should shop—to how to keep your mind active and alert as you age. So while you may have trained Skippy as a pup, let him begin to correct your bad habits to get you out of the dog house and onto happy trails to better living.

Don't get hooked on another quick-fix gimmick. Look around your house for the best personal trainer you can get—your best friend, Fluffy! Science proves it—having a furry, four-legged friend to walk at your heel and lick your face in the morning is great for your health! Having a dog in your life clearly improves your overall health, strengthens your heart, and reduces stress in your life. So give Max a pat on the head and a tummy scratch and let him show you the way to a healthier you.

LET YOUR DOG IMPROVE YOUR GENERAL HEALTH

If you do an Internet search on "physical fitness," your computer will suggest you visit over 35 million websites! While you're busy checking out the first 50 sites, your dog will be sitting next to you, wagging his tail, holding a partially chewed tennis ball, and asking for a nice game of fetch. "Not now," you say. "I'm busy trying to get in shape!" Now what's wrong with this picture?! You're trying to educate

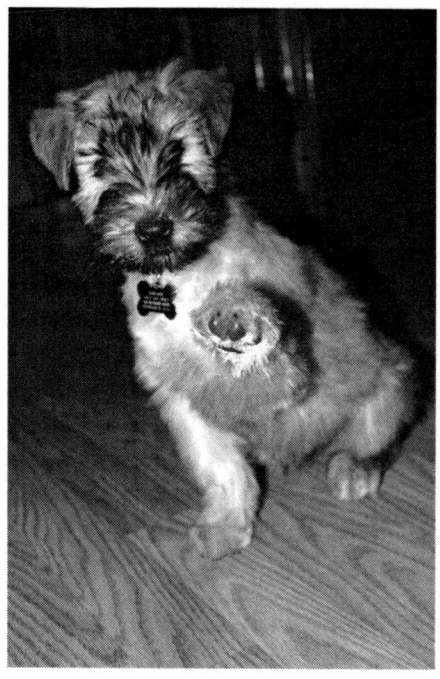

Take the pledge to follow your dog to better health.

your brain, while your dog knows you need to get up and change your behavior. Take advantage of the lessons you can learn from your furry friend to help gain a wealth of long-lasting good health rewards. Your dog can show you how to put all of that information you've been collecting in your intellect about good health to practical use.

When my doctor suggested I get a dog to help me get healthier, I assumed he was joking! Won't the extra work of caring for a dog just give me more stress? Sara P., Akron, OH

    I grew up with dogs—hunting dogs that provided us with pheasants and grouse for every holiday celebration. They also offered an accepting ear when times were tough, a ready jogging partner when running became a craze, and a soft pillow at the end of the day. Who knew my parents were providing both a friend and a guide to better health by having a dog in the house?

    Take this quiz to see if you know the health benefits that go along with owning a dog. Having a dog can help you:

- ☐ Lower your heart rate
- ☐ Decrease your blood pressure
- ☐ Reduce your blood triglyceride level
- ☐ Reduce your stress response
- ☐ Decrease excess weight
- ☐ Decrease loneliness

    If you chose every health benefit, you're absolutely right! Owning and exercising a dog helps improve your overall health, reduce your weight, and get your heart healthier (Voelker 2006). Interestingly, owning a dog seems to result in health benefits both from the increased physical activity involved with walking a dog, as well as the social support from simple companionship.

    If you've never owned a dog, don't despair—it's never too late to take that joyous plunge and begin to enjoy the benefits of a canine companion. Medical research shows that becoming a new dog owner results in both immediate and long-lasting health improvements (Serpell 1991). In a fascinating study, Dr. Serpell at the Department of Clinical Veterinary Medicine in Cambridge evaluated new pet owners and people without pets. While there was no change in minor health problems over six months among non-pet owners, dog owners experienced a 50 percent decrease in minor health problems after just one month of ownership. This benefit was maintained after six months. Interestingly, dog owners experienced a greater degree of health improvement than cat owners, and the benefits with dogs lasted longer than those seen with cats. Dog owners also experienced an increase in physical activity. On average, both future dog owners and non-pet owners walked an average of twice per week at the start of the study. This number decreased slightly over six months in the non-pet owners. After signing up with their four-legged trainers, dog owners experienced a substantial increase in the number of walks per week to nine per week after the first month and fourteen per week after six months.

Everyone knows that a regular physical exercise program can improve your health. Did you know that even walking 15 to 30 minutes per day can result in significant health benefits? Scientists consistently show that physical activity improves general health and mood. One study followed about one hundred sedentary women for six months after they were asked to start walking 90 minutes per week (Nies 2006). Most women did achieve the target walking goal. Seventy percent reported feeling more physically fit after walking, with almost half describing "more energy." Almost all of the women felt the walking made them "feel good," with mood improved in about one in five women and stress reduced in half.

Let your dog improve your general health:

- Increase daily walking
- Gain more energy
- Enjoy reduced stress
- Reduce minor health complaints

PUT ROVER IN CHARGE OF YOUR WEIGHT LOSS

As a skinny kid who ate everything in sight, I could never understand how people got overweight. After two kids and turning thirty and then forty, I soon learned that my metabolism had slowed and my clothes were beginning to shrink around my waist. (Okay, it was really the waist growing, but I was able to believe it was a faulty dryer until increasing to my third pants' size!) I soon learned that it wasn't just me—my friends and younger husband were also experiencing the same disturbing midlife change.

Since I've become a soccer mom, I run around constantly getting the kids to all of their activities. You'd think I'd be thin as a rail, but I've actually been gaining weight. Mary M., Turtle Creek, PA

Did you know that the average person begins to gain about one pound each year after age 35? So during midlife, you can expect to gain a whopping ten to fifteen pounds?! Yikes! And, you guessed it, this middle-aged gain usually lands right in our middle—around the belly, hips, and thighs. Fortunately, we don't have to take this "expected" aging expansion lying down, and our dogs can be the key to success.

Can a brisk dog walk really help? Won't I get more benefit from an aerobics class or jogging? Rich M., Jamaica, NY

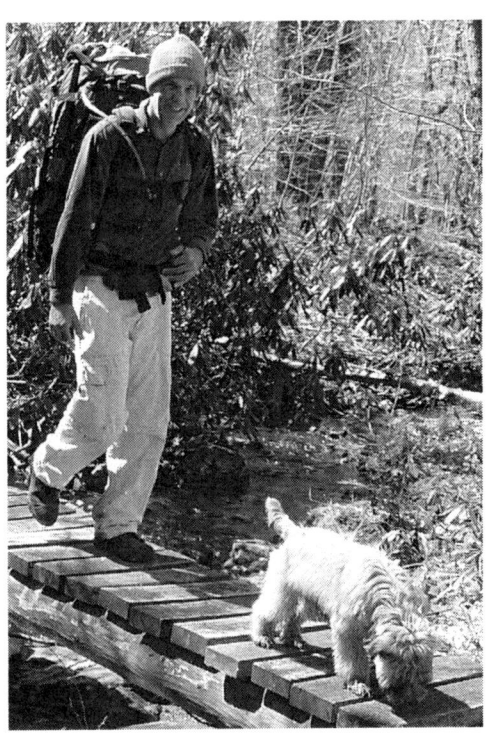

Take time out for a hike in the park.

Most of us have started many exercise programs—aerobics classes, Tae Bo, running programs—only to find we couldn't fit the programs into our routines. Many people believe that you'll only benefit from exercise and get your weight down if you exercise vigorously for at least 20 to 30 minutes. The good news is that we have a better chance of sticking with our exercise and losing weight by going for a couple short dog walks a day than from a once daily exercise program. Researchers at the University of Pittsburgh randomly assigned overweight adults to one of two exercise programs (Jakicic 1995). People in both programs were asked to exercise about 20 to 40 minutes a day on five days each week. One group was told they should break up their exercise minutes into several short exercise periods of about 10 minutes each. The other group was told to do one long fitness session each time they exercised. At the end of five months, the people using several short exercise periods to get in their daily work-out were exercising about 25 percent more days and for almost 20 percent longer in total duration compared with those needing to get their exercise done in a single, long session. People using the short exercise sessions also lost about 40 percent more weight! So you can probably get better exercise and weight loss by walking your dog for 10 minutes each walk two to four times a day than you will get from trying to stick to an exercise video.

The other great news is that you don't have to huff and puff to lose weight. Researchers in Texas compared weight loss among overweight, sedentary women who performed one of four exercise programs for one year (Chambliss 2005). The women all started walking 100 minutes per week at moderate intensity. This would be equivalent to a brisk walk where you're still able to talk while you're walking. If you can sing while you're walking, you need to increase your intensity level. Exercise duration was increased to 150 to 300 minutes per week and intensity varied from moderate to vigorous. Vigorous exercise would be where you would feel too winded or out of breath to carry on a conversation. At the end of the year, weight loss and heart benefits were similar in all of the exercise intensity groups. It was more important to walk at least 150 minutes per week than to use a vigorous intensity of exercise.

Let your dog help control your weight:

- Plan to walk your dog at least twice daily
- Plan to walk for at least 10 minutes per walk
- Try to walk a total of at least 150 minutes per week
- Walk briskly – you shouldn't be able to sing while you walk but you should still be able to chat comfortably

LET APOLLO STRENGTHEN YOUR HEART

Heart disease affects over 20 million Americans and is the number one killer for both men and women. There are a lot of factors that increase our risk for having heart disease or a heart attack. We can't change our genetics or our age, but we can reduce our risk from smoking, inactivity, obesity, high blood pressure, and high cholesterol with some hard work.

What risk factors do you have for heart disease?
- ☐ Previous heart attack or stroke
- ☐ Man older than age 45 or woman over 55
- ☐ High blood pressure (greater than 140/90)
- ☐ Diabetes
- ☐ Smoking
- ☐ More than 20 pounds overweight
- ☐ Exercise less than 30 minutes, 3 days per week
- ☐ High cholesterol
- ☐ Heart attack in dad or brother before age 55 OR mom or sister before age 65

If you checked 2 or more risk factors, be sure to talk to your doctor about ways to reduce your risk for heart disease. You'll probably receive encouragement to get more exercise to make your heart healthier and reduce excess weight. When your heart is stronger and healthier, your heart rate at rest and blood pressure are lower. This is encouraging news if there's a puppy in your house, since Buster can actually help improve your heart health.

Does owning a dog really make your heart healthier? Donna L., San Francisco, CA

A survey of the population in New South Wales concluded that dog walking could provide substantial benefits for reducing heart disease (Bauman 2001). Researchers predicted that if all dog owners began walking their dogs for 150 minutes per week, the overall population risk of heart disease would decrease by almost ten percent.

Dog owners tend to have healthier hearts with lower blood pressure and heart rates compared to non-owners (Anderson 1992, Allen 2002). In one comparison of risk factors for heart disease between pet owners and non-owners, both blood pressure and plasma triglycerides were decreased in the pet owners (Anderson 1992). Triglycerides are a type of fat in your bloodstream. Like cholesterol, high triglyercide levels also contribute to increased risk for heart disease. The authors speculated that better eating habits and exercise levels may have contributed to some of the lower heart disease risk factors among pet owners.

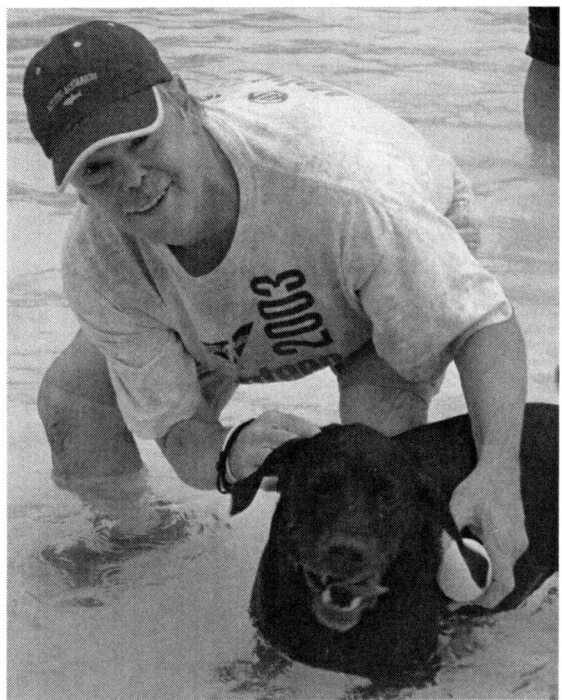

*Include a dog in your heart-healthy routine.
(Photo courtesy of Jillian Williams)*

I guess having Lady will help my heart because she encourages me to walk more. Joan P., Ithaca, NY

Dogs do more to help reduce stress on our hearts than just encourage us to get more active. In a unique experiment, 120 healthy adults were put into stressful situations with both mental stress from doing math calculations and physical stress (Allen 2002). Researchers measured heart response to stress by monitoring increased heart rate and blood pressure. Increases in heart rate and blood pressure show that the mental or physical stress is also causing stress on the heart. For both pet owners and non-pet owners, having their spouse or a supportive friend with them during the math test actually made their stress response worse. Having their pet with them during math calculations significantly *decreased* their stress response. Pet owners also made fewer errors in math calculations when their pet was in the room. The heart's response to physical stress was similarly improved in pet owners by having a pet nearby.

This response was also better with a pet than with a spouse or supportive friend. So the next time you need to balance your checkbook, talk with your teenager, or have dinner with your mother-in-law, make sure you have a four-legged friend nearby to help ease your stress level and help your heart.

People who have had heart attacks also do better if they have a dog to help them through their recovery. Researchers at Brooklyn College evaluated survival after having a heart attack (Friedmann 1995). Survival was substantially better for folks who had good social support—either human support or a dog. Within one year of having their heart attack, only one percent of dog owners died, compared with almost seven percent who didn't own dogs.

Dog owners have less heart disease risk due to:

- Increased exercise level
- Lower blood pressure
- Lower resting heart rate
- Lower stress response
- Better recovery after a heart attack

USE WALKING TO BOOST YOUR IMMUNE SYSTEM

Researchers at the University of Washington showed that regular, moderate intensity exercise (like brisk walking) helps improve your resistance to the common cold (Chubak 2006). In their study, 115 sedentary and overweight women were assigned to do either 45 minutes of moderate intensity exercise or 45 minutes of stretching 5 days weekly for one year. Before starting the study, women in both groups reported having the same number of colds. On average, women exercised about three and one-half days per week during the year of the study. Over the year, women doing moderate exercise experienced a modestly decreased risk of having a cold, while colds increased slightly in those doing only stretching. During the final three months of the study, the risk of colds was over three times higher among women doing just stretching compared with those doing daily aerobic exercise. So get exercising and give your tissue box a rest!

ALLOW PRINCESS TO PUT YOUR MIND AT EASE

Becoming more physically fit also improves your mood. Researchers at the University of Texas Southwestern Medical Center in Dallas studied physical fitness and emotional well-being in over 6,500 adults (Galper 2006). Physical fitness was judged by performance on a treadmill and reports of usual activity level. Physical inactivity and poor fitness levels were linked to poor emotional well-being and depression. As levels of physical activity increased, so did mental health.

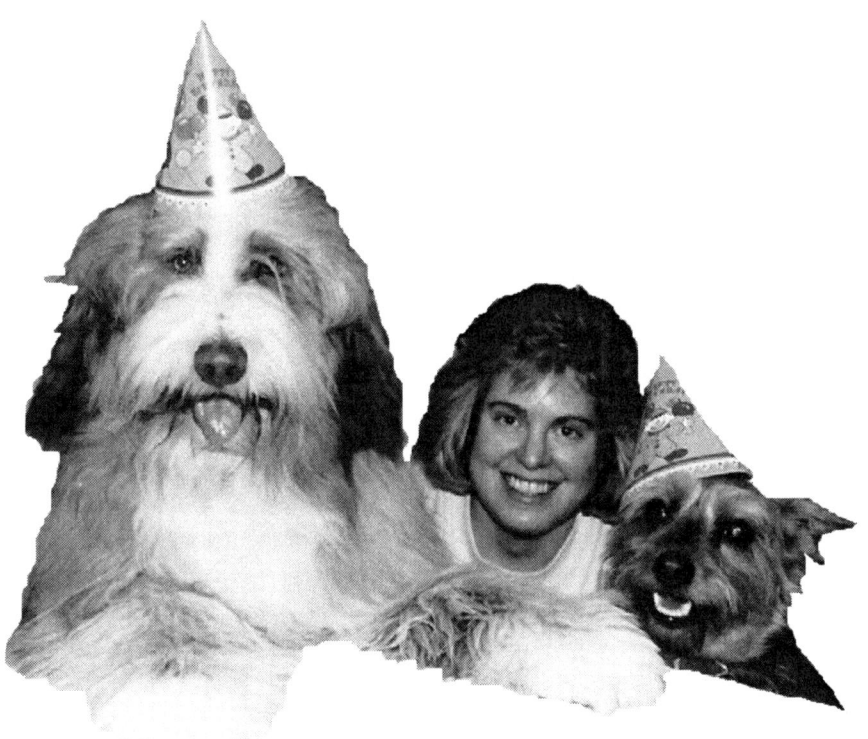

Celebrate life with the help of your furry friends. (Photo courtesy of Sherry Meininghaus)

Next time you're having a bad day, do a test. First, trying conducting your day just keeping to yourself. After about an hour of this, make a point of greeting people. Reach out to others with just simple phrases like, "Hello.

Have a nice day," "Nice to see you again," or "Isn't the weather awful today." Bet you'll notice that once you begin interacting with others, even for very short conversations, your mood will seem lighter and things won't seem as bad as they were when you were isolating yourself.

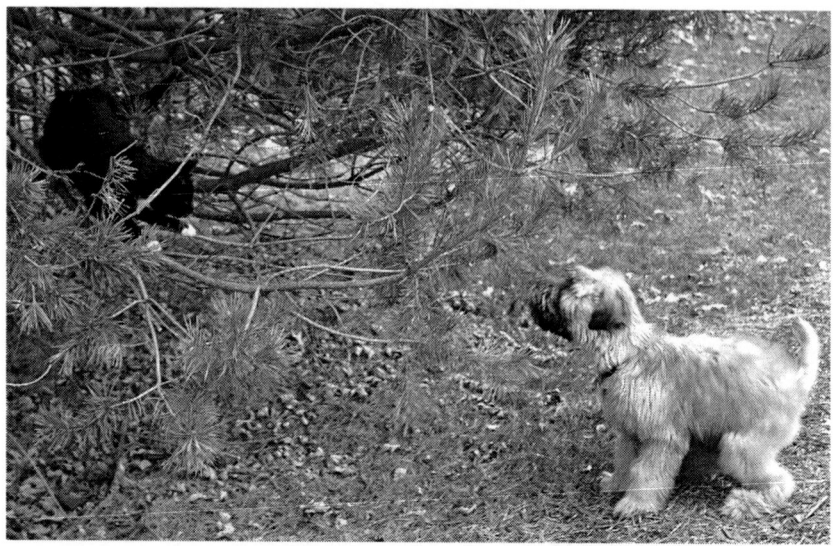

Wheatie's always excited to greet new friends. Take a lesson and greet your neighbors.

Having strong social interactions helps people feel connected with their community and reduces feelings of isolation, depression, and anxiety. When people move to a new community, develop health problems, or grow older, it's easy to lessen social interactions and feel more alone and distressed. Having a dog is a great way to increase your sphere of social interactions. In a study at the University of Warwick in the United Kingdom, psychologists monitored the number of social interactions in people if they were alone or accompanied by a dog (McNicholas 2000). People in the study were paired up with guide dogs trained to be inconspicuous and to avoid soliciting attention from others. People were encouraged to include dogs with their daily routine, such as taking their children to school, going to work at a university that permitted dogs, and riding public transportation. When a dog accompanied the person, there were over three times as many social encounters during these routine activities as when the person's routine was conducted with no dog. People had one-third more encounters with friends when they had a dog, with over twice as many encounters with acquaintances and over twenty times more encounters with strangers. Just having a dog at your side, therefore, widens your sphere of these important social interactions.

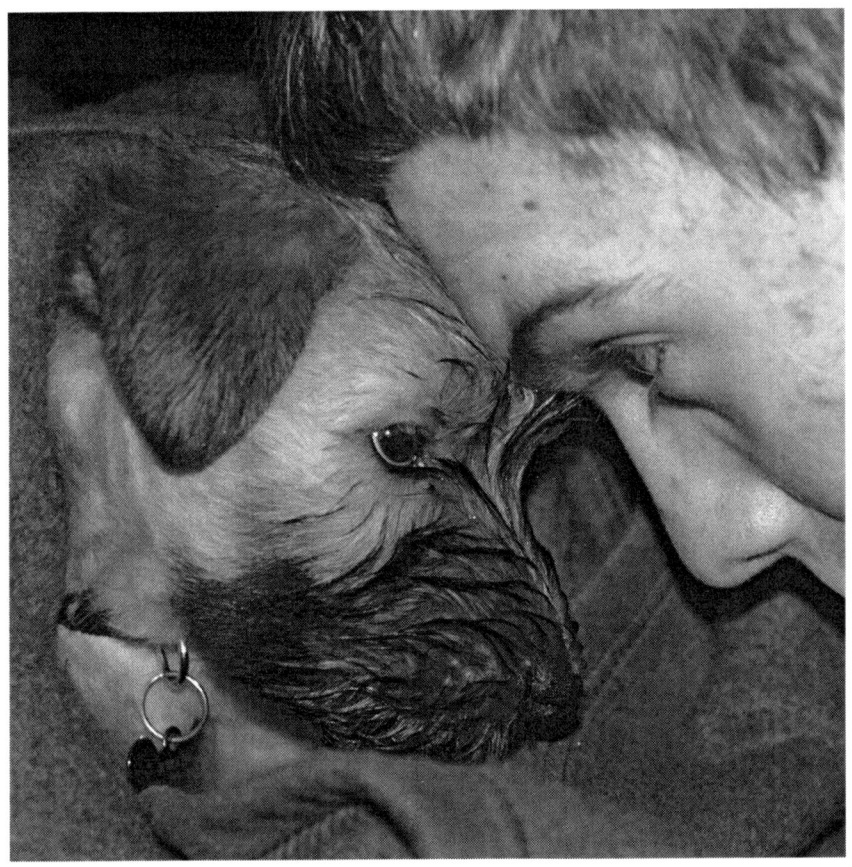

Get into your dog's head and learn some tips for better mental health.

KEEP YOUR TAIL WAGGING

I've been feeling down lately. I really have no interest in doing most of my chores, especially taking care of the dog. Will B., Cleveland, OH

Everyone feels blue now and then. Heck, I live in Pittsburgh and if the Steelers lose a game, the whole city plummets into the doldrums! Feeling blue is usually a mild and temporary feeling that goes away when situations improve. For some people, feeling temporarily blue can turn into depression. About one in ten people have problems with depression. When you're depressed, your mood can affect many aspects of your life—your appetite, sleep, interest in activities, and family life. It's hard to get motivated when you're feeling depressed. If you're just a bit down-in-the-dumps, becoming more physically active with your dog is a great way to chase those blues away. If your mood problem is more severe or you have depression, it's important to see your doctor, get a diagnosis, and start treatment.

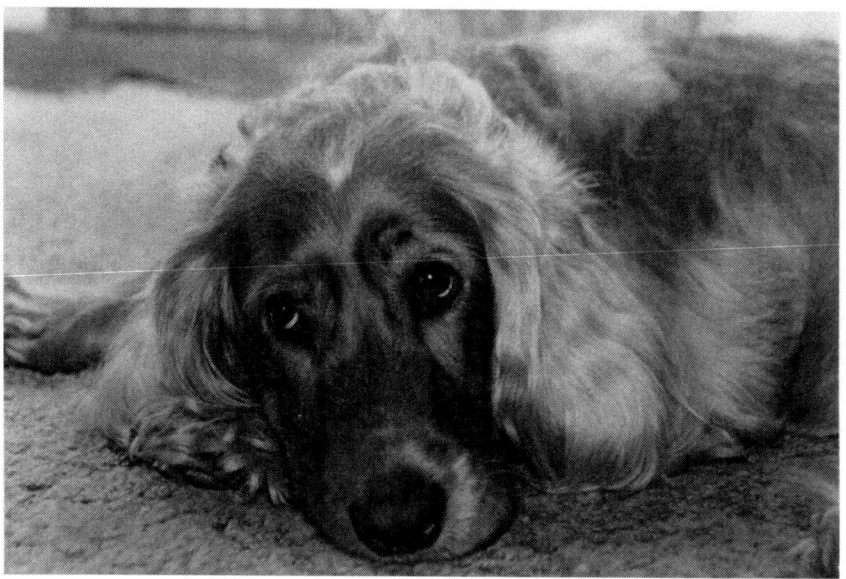

Take action if you begin to feel blue.

There are several good depression screening tests on the Internet:
- http://www.depression-screening.org/
- http://www.med.nyu.edu/psych/screens/depres.html
- http://allpsych.com/tests/diagnostic/index.html

Take this quiz to see if depression may be a problem for you:
☐ Do you frequently feel sad, irritable, or quick to anger?
☐ Have you stopped enjoying your hobbies and other

things you used to enjoy?
- ☐ Do you feel guilty or hopeless or worry too much?
- ☐ Do you feel out of energy or just prefer to sit alone more than usual?
- ☐ Have you stopped participating in social events with your family or friends?
- ☐ Are you sleeping too long or having trouble getting to sleep?
- ☐ Have you experienced a 10-pound change in your weight that you didn't intend to have?
- ☐ Do you have thoughts of suicide or death?

If you answered yes to the last question or at least two of the other questions, talk to your doctor. These feelings can be symptoms of depression. They can also be caused by other health problems, like anemia, thyroid disease, medication side effects, or other medical conditions.

DON'T LET WORRYING TAKE OVER

My husband is always badgering me to stop worrying. Now I'm worrying about when he comes home and asks if I spent the day worrying. Linda J., Allison Park, PA

Everyone worries now and then—will my son thrive in that faraway college, will I get this project completed by the deadline, is that mole on my arm something serious? Some people, however, seem to worry more than others. If you're a worrier, your family, co-workers, and friends probably tell you to stop worrying. And they are right—worrying is bad for your health. In one survey, people who worried for at least one month were more likely to have mental distress, like depression, anxiety, and panic disorder. They were also more likely to have physical diseases, like heart disease and even cancer (Noyes 2005). Getting busy with caring for your dog's needs and playing physical games with Tucker, like fetch or tug-of-war, can be a great way to relieve tension and help focus your attention away from your worries.

If you can't stop worrying or feeling anxious affects your life or your family, you may have an anxiety disorder. About ten percent of people develop an anxiety disorder. If you think you might have an anxiety disorder, see your doctor for a diagnosis and treatment. Worrying and feeling anxious are exhausting and stressful and there are many effective treatments to relieve these symptoms.

There are several good Internet anxiety screening tools:

- http://www.med.nyu.edu/psych/screens/
- http://allpsych.com/tests/diagnostic/index.html
- http://psychcentral.com/quizzes/anxiety.htm

Take this quiz to see if anxiety may be a problem for you:
- ☐ Do you frequently worry?
- ☐ Do you have trouble feeling relaxed? When you try to relax does your mind start racing about small problems?
- ☐ Do you have difficulty sitting still or concentrating?
- ☐ Are you afraid to make a decision and tend to second guess your choices?
- ☐ Do groups of people make you nervous or do you avoid social situations?
- ☐ Do you have problems with your stomach or bowel habits?

If you answered yes to at least two of these questions, talk to your doctor. These feelings can be symptoms of an anxiety disorder. They can also be caused by other health problems, like low blood sugar, thyroid disease, medication side effects, or other medical conditions.

TAKE A BITE OUT OF STRESS

I feel like I spend the day racing around and getting nothing accomplished. When the family is finally together at the end of the day, I'm too stressed out to relax and enjoy them. Nora S., Chicago, IL

Most everyone leads full and busy lives. Years ago, we thought having more technology would make our lives easier and more relaxed. Unfortunately, the world of instant messaging, fax machines, and emails seems to have just sped up our lives. We try to fit more and more activities and chores into each day. When I was in grade school, kids played softball after school or maybe attended Scouts once a week. Now, we rush our kids to almost daily after-school activities—music practice, soccer, karate classes, academic seminars, etc. If there's an extra minute in the day, we'll probably find a way to fill it up. This has led most people to feel stressed—both at work and at home.

Stress is important because it causes mental distress and also can aggravate other medical problems. Stress often triggers headaches, stomach aches and diarrhea, elevated blood pressure, sleep trouble, and mood disturbances. Stress can also strain your heart. Take the following quiz to see if you are susceptible to developing physical symptoms from mental stress:

- ☐ Do you have trouble finding someone to share problems with?
- ☐ Have you stopped attending to your spiritual needs?
- ☐ Have you stopped making time for your hobbies?
- ☐ Do you frequently skip meals?
- ☐ Do you drink more than 2 cups of caffeinated beverages daily?
- ☐ Do you regularly smoke or drink alcohol?
- ☐ Are you overweight?
- ☐ Do you frequently sleep less than 7 hours per night?
- ☐ Do you usually exercise less than every other day?
- ☐ Do you worry about doing a good job at work?
- ☐ Do you worry that you won't be able to pay your bills?

If you checked four or more boxes, you're at risk for stress aggravating physical problems. The more of these boxes that you checked, the more vulnerable you are to developing physical symptoms when exposed to stress.

While there are shelves of paperbacks at most bookstores claiming to have the key to improving your mood and relieving stress in your life, don't forget to turn to Shadow to decrease psychological distress. Interacting with a dog is a great stress reliever, resulting in relaxation and reduced anxiety (Wilson 1991). In one study, anxiety was measured in college students. Anxiety levels dropped by about ten percent when the students were allowed to pet and talk to a dog (Wilson 1991). Dogs also provide a buffer against bad health effects from stress (Siegel 1990). Dog owners are less likely to need attention for medical complaints during times of stress compared with non-owners.

My daughter picked a long-haired dog. So now I need to visit the groomer each month. This has just added extra stress to my already-busy life. Susan K., Wheeling, WV

It's funny how we have no problem arranging time for others to get some fun and pampering—we take our kids to play groups, an elderly relative to the beauty salon, and our dog to the groomer. We usually forget, however, to schedule time to pamper ourselves. Watch your dog and learn from her example.

Dog owners often take the dog to the groomer once a month for a full pampering—nails, teeth, and hair. While the dog's spending a day being groomed and fussed over, the owner will dash off to complete a list of necessary chores, dashing from store to store or chore to chore. What if we decided to give ourselves a day of pampering each month? We might spend a day relaxing in the tub, giving ourselves a pedicure, getting our hair styled. At the end of this pampering, we might come out looking like our dogs. Have you ever noticed the dogs as they leave the grooming salon? Even the dogs who fight going in and

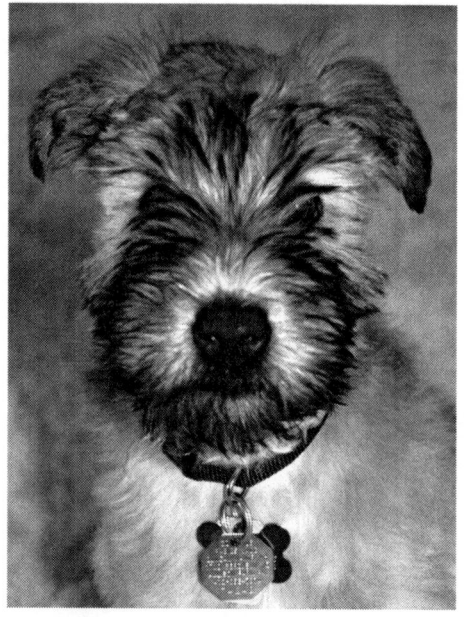

Take time to pamper yourself and feel as cute as a puppy.

give groomers a hard time leave with a new lift in their step, with a look of "Oh yeah. I'm beautiful. Hey, not the hair—don't muss up the hair!"

SCHEDULE A BREAK

After a hard day, I come home, race to get chores done and yell at the kids. My lazy dog looks at me, sighs, and just plops down for a nap! Anna T., Maine, NY

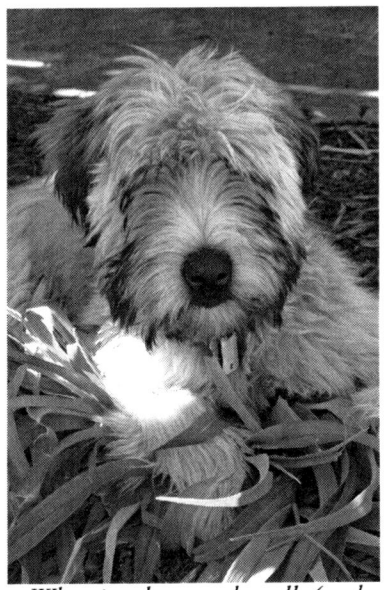

Wheatie relaxes and smells (and sometimes eats!) the flowers.

Too many of us face stress and a hectic schedule by increasing the chaos and trying to cram even more activities into an already over-scheduled routine. Next time you're racing around, take a break and look at Lucky—he's probably sprawled out in the middle of the floor. Lucky's the picture of total relaxation. Instead of taunting, "It's nice *someone* around here gets to take a break," consider adopting his style. You probably don't want to collapse in the middle of the kitchen, but you might try practicing some relaxation techniques (see below).

Practice the following exercises daily until you have mastered them. Then use them before confronting stressful situations or at the end of a stressful day. You can perform many of these while standing in the shower or in a long line at the grocery store, waiting in traffic, or brushing Ginger. You might wish to listen to soothing music while you relax:

- SLOW YOUR RHYTHM—DEEP BREATHING RELAXATION
  o Sit in a stiff chair with your hands in your lap and feet on the floor. Close your eyes. Take a deep breath. Feel both your chest and abdomen expand. Hold for three seconds. Then slowly exhale over five seconds by softly saying the

word "relax" out loud five times. Wait for a count of three, then repeat. Repeat ten times.
- **KEEP TENSION FROM YOUR BODY—PROGRESSIVE MUSCLE RELAXATION**
  o Sit in a stiff chair with your hands in your lap and feet on the floor. Close your eyes. Practice tightening the muscles in your feet and hold for ten seconds. Then relax the muscles in your feet for ten seconds. Work your way up the body, alternatively contracting and relaxing muscles. Move from the muscles in your feet to your legs, your buttocks, your abdomen, your arms, your shoulders, your neck, and your face. Pay attention to how each muscle feels when it's tight and then relaxed.
  o Next time you're beginning to feel stressed, make a note of which muscles feel tight. Then take a deep breath, close your eyes, and practice helping those tight muscles feel relaxed. You'll feel the tension slip away.
- **CHANGE THE WAY YOU THINK ABOUT PROBLEMS —COGNITIVE RESTRUCTURING**
  o Cognitive restructuring involves changing your internal thoughts and the messages you tell yourself from negative to positive. It's easy to think negative thoughts like, "I'll never get this project completed!" or "I'll never lose weight. I guess I'm just destined to be three sizes too big!" or "When will this dog ever be housebroken—it's hopeless!" The more we hear these negative views, the more we begin to believe them and the more depressed, anxious, and stressed we become.
  o We tell our dogs positive messages all the time: "What a good girl!", "You're so precious", "Such a pretty doggie." Cognitive restructuring involves using these same kinds of positive messages on ourselves.
  o Make a point of giving positive messages to yourself. Turn your negative messages into something positive. When faced with a looming deadline, say, "You'll succeed. You did a good job getting that project done on time last month." When struggling with a weight loss program, tell yourself, "I've been doing a good job sticking to my walking program. And I haven't gained back the three pounds I lost last month." When discovering an unwelcome "treasure" left by Buster, remind yourself, "He'll eventually get

housebroken. It's been a week between accidents, so they're less frequent than they used to be."
- **LOOSEN YOUR MUSCLES—STRETCHING EXERCISES**
  - Sit on a stiff chair with your hands in your lap and both feet on the floor.
  - Close your eyes and breathe slowly.
  - Slowly tip your right ear to your right shoulder. Hold for five seconds. Now tip your left ear to your left shoulder. Hold for five seconds. Now bend your chin to chest. Hold for five seconds. Now tip your face up toward the ceiling. Hold for five seconds. Repeat five times. Return to the starting position.
  - Raise both arms over your head, reaching with your finger tips toward the ceiling. Don't arch your back. Hold for five seconds. Then reach both arms out to the side, as though you're trying to pull each arm away from your body. Hold for five seconds. Then reach both arms in front of your chest, with your fingers trying to reach as far away from your chest as possible. Hold for five seconds. Repeat five times. Return to the starting position.
  - Straighten both knees, lifting your feet off of the floor. Pull your toes back toward your knees. Feel a stretch behind your knee in your calves. Hold for five seconds. Now point your toes away from your knees. Feel the stretch in the top of your feet. Hold for five seconds. Repeat moving your toes toward and away from you, holding each position for five seconds, for a total of five repetitions. Then place your feet back on the floor. Rest for three seconds. Then repeat three times.

Once you're practicing these techniques, watch your dog. I bet you'll notice that he often takes a big sigh or a long full body stretch during the day. And when you hear yourself praising Rascal, "Good boy! What a good dog. You're just so sweet," remember to use these same kinds of positive phrases on yourself. Your dog benefits from hearing positive phrases about himself and you will, too.

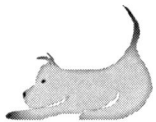

MAKE DOG WALKS A TOP PRIORITY

If you can't find time take three short 10-minute walks with your dog each day, you're too busy and you need to streamline your routine. Look at ways to simplify your life and avoid over-scheduling yourself.

- Remember you're not responsible for everyone's happiness and needs. Don't try to rescue your family members or friends from every difficult or frustrating situation. Facing adversity builds character. So give them emotional support, then back off and let them struggle to find solutions and succeed. When Junior's working on his English paper, don't hover behind him giving suggestions. Take Duke for a walk. When you come back, help proofread the paper. Junior's learned more and you got in a walk.

- Ask family members to help with household chores. Ask Sister to fold the laundry while you and your toddler walk the dog. When you're out walking, you won't have to watch her roll her eyes and hear her complain about how unfair you are. And when you come back, a chore will be checked off your list and you were able to walk.

- Only volunteer for one or two activities. You don't need to do it all.

- Break big projects down into several smaller tasks. Tackle one small task at a time.

- Keep regular meal times. And never eat on the run.

- Keep regular sleep times. Don't stay up late finishing chores; they'll wait until morning.

- Avoid excess caffeine, alcohol, and nicotine.

Let your dog help your emotional state:

- Keep your dog nearby during times of stress
- Use physical play with your dog to release tension
- Take your dog's cue and relax during times of stress

TAKE PRIDE IN BEING AN "OLD DOG"

Remember when you were a kid and adults in their 40's were "really old." In a blink of an eye, 40 didn't look so old anymore and before you knew it, you were talking about folks who were "only 70." While we may begin to look a bit worn and old to young kids, Honey will always look at you like you're the perfect playmate—regardless of your age. Luckily, you can enjoy terrific benefits from a friendship with your pooch whether you're six, sixteen, or sixty-plus.

Older adults can also achieve comparable benefits from dog ownership as are seen in younger folks. For example, similar to studies in younger adults, a survey of adults 60 years and older showed that dog owners walk more than non-owners and have lower blood triglyceride levels (Dembicki 1996). Pet owners are also more likely to remain active than non-owners (Raina 1999).

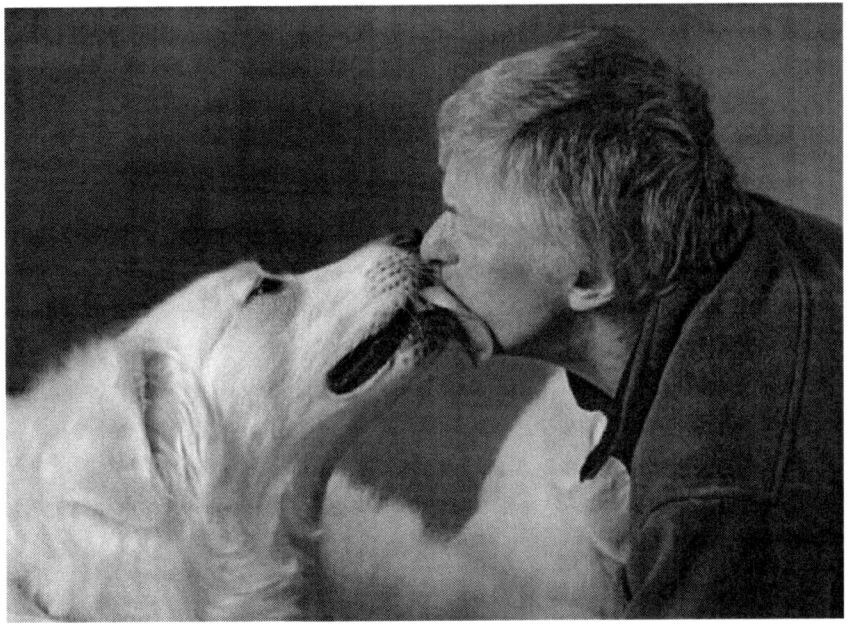

Dogs provide health benefits for all ages. (Photo courtesy of Joyce Arnowitz)

My mother lives alone and wants a dog for companionship. I have enough trouble worrying about her, let alone a dog, too! **Marion K., Daytona Beach, FL**

Senior dog owners enjoy improved physical activity, spending more time outdoors (Siegel 1990, Raina 1999) and walking about twice as often as non-owners (Rogers 1993). Older dog owners also experience less stress and loneliness, better nutrition, and a stronger focus on the present (Rogers 1993). Seniors in mobile home parks in central California were asked to take typical daily walks (Rogers 1993). Dog owners walked once with their dogs and once without their dogs. Walkers carried a hidden tape recorder to monitor conversations during these walks. Non-owners tended to talk about health problems and the past, while dog owners were more likely to talk about their dogs and present day events. Walking with the dog increased the number of conversations about the dog. Walking with the dog also promoted light, social banter with the dog during the walk when not speaking with other people. Therefore, walking with a dog tends to promote a healthier focus on the present and off of troubling health concerns in seniors.

When considering adding a dog to a senior's home:

- Make sure the senior wants to have a dog
- Be sure the senior can care for a dog—physically, mentally, and financially
- Arrange for plans to care for the dog if the senior becomes unable to keep the dog
- Avoid toy breeds and stubborn dogs like terriers that may get underfoot and precipitate falls
- Consider older dogs that are already trained and less active

Seniors can get benefits from dog companionship by volunteering at animal shelters or having pet therapy visits.

Dogs help seniors by:

- Providing consistent companionship
- Increasing physical activity
- Doubling walking time
- Helping seniors focus on the here-and-now
- Reducing concerns about health problems

Chapter 2.

Eat Like a Dog

Janice had struggled with weight since the birth of her second child. At each annual check-up her doctor had commented that she'd put on an extra five or ten pounds. Every time she got on the scale, she felt discouraged and embarrassed. This year, Janice took her four-year-old golden Lab to the vet for her yearly shots and was shocked when the vet walked in announcing, "Honey really put on some winter weight this year!" Fortunately for Janice, the usual denials she used when the doctor tried to counsel her about her own weight didn't work on the vet and she decided both she and Honey would commit to losing those extra pounds.

Obesity is a national problem, affecting nearly one in four adults in the United States (CDC 2006). Obesity is not just a US problem. A recent report from England estimates that in 2010, one in three men and one in four women will be obese (O'Dowd 2006). In China, one in five adults is overweight or obese (Wu 2006).

Just as human obesity is on the rise, so is dog obesity. Studies show that about one in three dogs is overweight (McGreevy 2005, Colliard 2006). In an interesting study, scientists in Germany evaluated the owners of obese and normal weight dogs (Kienzle 1998). Obese dogs received less exercise and were rewarded with food when they sought attention. Although both normal and obese dogs received similar food portions at meal times, the overweight dogs were more "humanized" in their eating and lifestyle habits. The researchers noticed that the overweight dogs were treated like "fellow humans," rather than companion dogs. Dogs living a typical dog life tended to be in better shape and of normal weight. The authors concluded that dogs needed to be treated like dogs rather than another family member. You might also consider that changing the owner's eating habits to be more "dog-like" might also help him lead a dog's life and get into better shape.

Take the following eating habits quiz. Check any behavior that you typically do three or more times a week:
- ☐ Skip at least one meal a day
- ☐ Eat snacks between meals
- ☐ Eat on the run, in the car, or while doing work
- ☐ Eat while relaxing, reading, or watching television
- ☐ Finish leftovers right after a meal so they don't go to waste
- ☐ Drink less than 10 cups of water a day
- ☐ Try new snack items offered at your grocery store

If you checked any of these, you need to improve your eating habits. Think about Jake—does he usually skip meals, avoid drinking lots of water, or eat when he's playing? If he's fit and healthy, he won't do any of these. If he's getting lots of between meal snacks, you'll need to watch your own snacking and also stop spoiling his appetite! Follow Jake's natural eating pattern and you'll find you're eating like a dog and avoiding bad eating habits.

SWITCH TO A SMALLER DOG DISH

I've been watching what I eat, but still don't seem to lose any weight. Barb R., Steubenville, OH

Do you remember when the only size French fries that came with your take-out hamburger was the little size that's now used only in kiddie meals? Part of the reason Americans are getting bigger is because their food portions are expanding. For example, the United States Department of Agriculture recommends eating 5½ ounces of meat daily for the average adult eating a typical 2000 calorie per day diet; however, the largest hamburgers sold at popular fast-food chains are 8 to 12 ounces (Young 2007). One 12-ounce burger would be the recommended portion for two full days—not one meal! And burgers are just the tip of the iceberg. Researchers from the Department of Nutrition at the University of North Carolina evaluated average portion sizes for a wide variety of foods over two decades (Nielsen 2003). Portion sizes increased for every food surveyed, except for pizza. See Table 1 comparing serving sizes for a variety of common foods in 1977 and in 1996. So a hamburger, fries, and cola in 1996 would result in 214 more calories than the "same" meal ordered in 1977. You'd need to walk your dog at a moderate pace for an extra hour to burn off those extra calories!

Table 1. *Portion sizes have increased over times*

Food Category	Average Portion Size in Ounces		Extra Calories in 1996
	1977	1996	
Salty snacks	1.0	1.6	93
Desserts	4.5	4.8	41
Soft drinks	13.1	19.9	49
Fruit drinks	11.3	15.1	50
French fries	3.1	3.6	68
Hamburgers	5.7	7.0	97

So have we gotten smarter about our portions since the 90's? You can predict from the increase in obesity since then that the answer is a resounding NO! Recently, researchers at Colorado and San Diego State Universities compared actual portions selected by college students with standard portion sizes (Burger 2007). This comparison is highlighted in Table 2. You can see from the Table that most food items were consumed in higher portions than what is considered to be "normal" portion sizes by most of the students. Snack foods and cola were consumed in portions twice as big as the standard sizes. And double the portion means double the calories—so you'll need twice as much exercise.

Table 2. *Comparison of standard portion sizes with actual portions eaten by college students*

Food	Standard portion size	Actual portion size selected	Percentage of students exceeding the standard portion size
Peanuts	30 grams	58 grams	98%
Rice	140 grams	198 grams	76%
Chocolate candies	40 grams	97 grams	84%
Tortilla chips	30 grams	58 grams	78%
Cold cereal	30 grams	54 grams	94%
Macaroni and cheese	132 grams	188 grams	43%
Cola	240 mL	464 mL	80%

It's not just eating out that's the problem. Similar increases in portion sizes occur in food consumed in the home or at restaurants (Nielsen 2003). So we can't just blame restaurant and cafeteria managers, since we're seeing the same increases in foods we prepare for ourselves at home. We need to re-educate ourselves about appropriate portion sizes. One serving size of each of the foods below can be easily visualized:

- Meat = computer mouse
- Pasta = ½ baseball
- Cereal = small individual box
- Cheese = 9-volt battery
- Peanut butter = ping pong ball
- Chips, crackers, or popcorn = one handful

An easy way to limit portions is to use smaller dishes and bowls. Try using dessert bowls for your breakfast cereal and dessert plates for your regular meal plates. Your dish will look fuller, so you won't feel like you're skimping on meals.

Also, limit the size of your snacks. Don't eat your snacks right out of a large bag. Even most smaller snack bags contain more than one serving. Use the small "fun-size" snack bags offered for Halloween trick-or-treaters or get some resealable plastic snack size bags and make your own snack sizes for your favorite treats. I admit it—I LOVE chocolate! When I open a candy bar, I actually get the most enjoyment from the first, mouth-watering bite. You know, the one where you sigh and say, "This is SO delicious!" By the time I've had my fifth mouthful, or half dozen cookies, that thrill is gone and then I'm sort of chewing just to keep my jaws busy. Using small, "fun-size" snacks gives you the pleasure of the snack without the guilt of stuffing yourself.

Unlike human treats, dog treats are typically fairly small. At our house, I break the usual small dog treats in half. Since my dog's in training, I really like to limit the total quantity of treats by keeping each individual treat very small. My husband is still amazed that Wheatie will snap to attention for a reward about the size of a mini chocolate chip. I've tried to learn from his response to treats. He seems to get just as much pleasure from the tiny treat as he does from a large treat when I am too lazy to break it into pieces. Try making your treats tiny, and you'll probably discover you're just as satisfied with the yummy taste as a full belly of sugary, fatty treats.

KEEP REGULAR FEEDING TIMES

I don't know how I gain weight. I never have time to sit down for a meal. Bob T., Pittsburgh, PA

If you skip meals, you're not alone. Busy lifestyles have led many people to opt for meals on the run. About ten percent of people intentionally skip meals, because they believe skipping meals will help them lose weight (Kruger 2004). I don't have to tell you Buster's views on meal skipping. He'd tell you the same thing you heard growing up, "I don't want to hear you're too busy or want to do something else. It's dinner time, so sit down and eat this meal I prepared for you!"

Researchers at the University of Massachusetts Medical School evaluated eating patterns in almost 500 adults (Ma 2003). They found that people skipping breakfast were four and a half times more likely to be obese than those who regularly ate breakfast. It also mattered where they ate. People who frequently ate breakfast or dinner away from home were also more likely to be obese. When people ate breakfast or lunch away from home, the meal tended to have more calories, more fat, and less healthy fiber. This study suggests that better weight control will be achieved if you eat regular meals at home, rather than skipping meals and catching meals on the run.

So schedule regular feeding times and stick to them. You probably wouldn't think of tossing Lassie in the back seat with a bowl of kibble, but you may think nothing's wrong with eating your breakfast in the car on the way to work or driving the kids to school. Just like Lassie, you need to sit down for a regular meal at home. It's healthier for you. And, if you're trying to lose weight, it's a much better diet strategy than skipping meals or eating on the run.

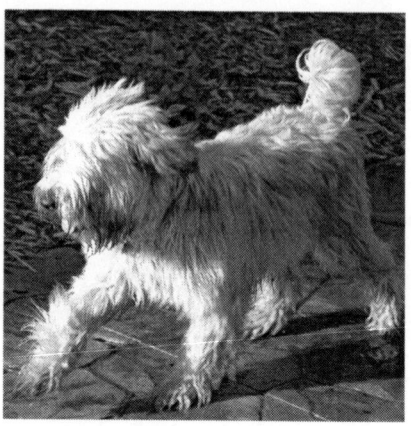

Wheatie doesn't eat on the run, and neither should you.

Part of the reason I skip meals is because I catch myself snacking so much between meals. I have to cut calories somewhere. Megan I., Monroeville, PA

Skipping meals is a common problem. About 40 percent of adults skip at least one meal over a two-day period (Howarth 2006). Although you might think breakfast is the most commonly missed meal, people are actually most likely to skip lunch (Howarth 2006). The problem with skipping meals is that meal skipping usually results in in-between meal snacking. In one survey, people ate an average of two snacks each day (Howarth 2006). In this same survey, people eating three meals a day tended to be normal weight, while those eating more often than three meals a day were overweight.

I've found that I have several times a day where, like clockwork, I become famished. It really doesn't seem to matter if I ate a good meal one, two, or even half an hour before my scheduled time. The clock strikes and I get hunger pangs. For me, the times are 10 a.m., 2 p.m., and 5:30 p.m. I've adjusted breakfast and lunch to coincide with the first two times, but am unable to eat an early dinner since my kids aren't home from sport's practice until around 7:30 p.m. Before Wheatie came along, I'd start preparing dinner around 5:30 p.m. and would gobble down more than a meal's worth of food before the preparation was complete. When dinner was finally served, I'd feel too embarrassed to admit I'd already eaten a meal and a half. Being raised by

Depression Era parents, I couldn't leave food on my plate, so my one and one-half dinners would expand into two and a half dinners and I'd need to loosen my belt another notch.

Now I try to schedule a walk when one of these hunger pangs starts. Wheatie has yet to refuse to go walking. Sometimes I get a look of "Again? Didn't we just come back from a walk?" But after a sigh, he gets up and happily trots to the door. By the time we're back, my appetite has usually calmed down and I can wait the short time before the family sits down for a real meal.

KENNEL UP FOR FOOD

I've tried to limit between-meal snacking. But, before I know it, I'm munching on peanut butter crackers, pretzels, and other snacks I have for the kids in the pantry. Jeanne L., Norman, OK

I grew up with dogs joining the family for meal time, a welcome treat for a little girl who wanted to dispose of gristle and fat from meat, as well as least favorite foods. As an adult, however, I don't appreciate dogs begging at meal time. So we ask our terrier to "kennel up" whenever food comes out. Try using this technique for snack times, as well. If you religiously kennel Lucky every time you get out even the smallest snack, you'll soon find you're snacking less often. Kenneling the dog before you eat makes you take a few minutes break to determine if you really need a dish of ice cream or a handful of cookies an hour before dinner. If you're a frequent snacker, this will become obvious when you're regularly asking your dog to go to his kennel so you can nibble something. Kenneling your dog with every snack can help make you more aware of your own bad eating behavior.

DON'T GRAZE WHEN YOU'RE BORED

I sometimes don't even realize how much I snack. When I sit down to watch television or open the mail, I just start nibbling. Larry T., Los Angeles, CA

Don't snack when you're bored. When I'm bored, I'll usually plop myself in front of some mindless television show, and start snacking on anything and everything. I don't really pay attention to what I'm eating; it's more of a way to keep hands and mouth busy. This behavior is completely the opposite of what a dog does when he's bored.

Every now and then, I'm too wrapped up in work and Wheatie spends much of the day just lying around. He clearly looks bored and jumps up excitedly whenever I get up for a drink or trip to the bathroom. He also wanders over to his food dish, sniffs the leftovers from breakfast, and passes them by. When he's bored, his solution is usually to go outside and dig a hole or find some other entertainment, like catching rain drops or chasing butterflies. Model your response to boredom after your dog. Don't munch. Get active.

So when you're bored, don't look to the kitchen. Look for a physical activity—go for a walk, play ball with your dog, do some jumping jacks, or take a shower. The physical exertion will act as a stress reliever for your mind and put you in a better frame of mind to have a positive attitude to find something interesting or entertaining.

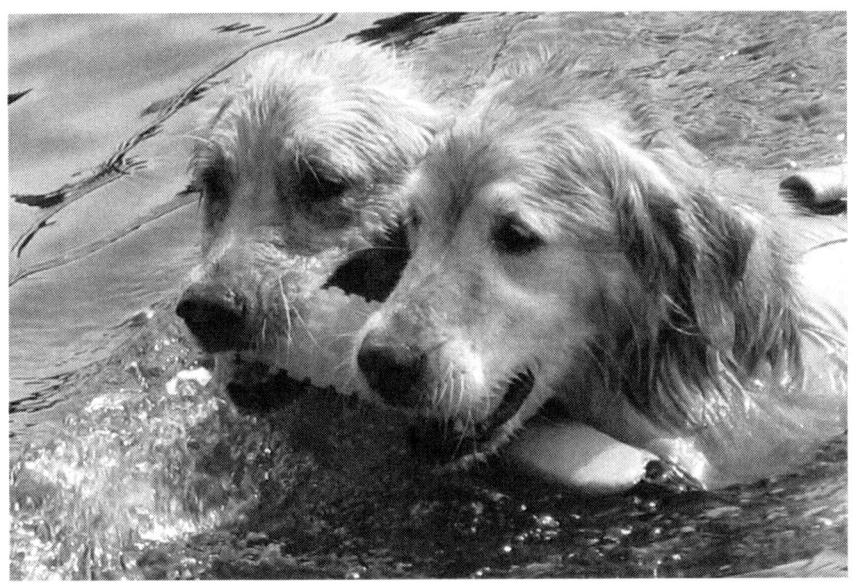

When you're sitting around and bored, reach for your dog's leash or a Frisbee rather than a bag of chips. (Photo courtesy of Susan Borzelleca)

DON'T EAT TABLE SCRAPS

I'm good about reducing my portion sizes, but when I'm cleaning up the dinner dishes, I find myself nibbling the leftovers on my kids' plates. Mary H., Wexford, PA

Growing up, I was required to finish the food served on my plate. We all heard the same phrases: Waste not, want not. Starving children across the world. As an adult, it's easy to remember these reminders and hard not to heed them. In today's super-sized meal world, portion sizes provided in restaurants and even at home are often too big. So it's very tempting to gobble down these leftovers to "clean the plate." As moms, it's also tempting to nibble down those leftover French fries, the half of a sandwich, handful of cookie bites, or (my favorite) pizza crusts remaining on Junior's plate. Next time that uneaten jelly donut on the breakfast tray seems to be calling you, stop and think about how you handle leftovers for Buster.

Your vet has probably cautioned you not to give your dog table scraps. "Dog food is for dogs and people food for people." You shouldn't give your dog table scraps because it's not healthy for him—he already gets enough nutrition and calories from his regular dog food. You wouldn't encourage Lucky to jump up on your kitchen table and finish the scraps off of everyone's plates. Don't do the same thing yourself. And the next time you're tempted to finish that half eaten candy bar leftover in Bobby's lunchbox, remember Lucky and toss it in the trash. You probably wouldn't think about gobbling Murphy's leftover kibble. Don't eat leftover human kibble either.

Eat like a dog

- Don't overfill your food dish – watch portion sizes
- Schedule regular feeding times
- Don't eat when you're bored
- Don't eat table scraps

KEEP YOUR WATER DISH FULL

Whenever I start a new exercise program, I finish exercising and eat, eat, EAT! I can't lose weight because exercising makes me eat too much.
Melissa R., Zelienople, PA

After beginning a new exercise program, many people feel the need to eat something immediately after working out. When that something is a half dozen donuts or a bag of chocolate chip cookies, it's hard to see how exercising will help you lose weight. Actually, this after-exercise craving is usually not a desire for food, but a craving for water replenishment. Next time, drink eight to twelve ounces of water at the end of an exercise session, and you'll probably curb that urge to eat more calories than you burned.

Your dog has already learned the importance of hydration before, during, and after exercise. Dogs will usually accept drinks throughout their exercise. When they return home from a romp, they run to the water bowl, not the food dish. Like your dog, it's important that you keep your "water dish" full and drink from it frequently.

Do you know how much you should drink each day? Take this quiz to see if you can spot the correct answer about staying hydrated:

- ☐ You only need to drink 3-5 beverages each day, unless you're exercising heavily.
- ☐ People who drink 8-10 beverages a day put an unnecessary strain on their kidneys.
- ☐ It's okay to be mildly dehydrated, as long as you still urinate a couple of times a day.
- ☐ Restricting water is a great way to drop several pounds in a few days.

If you said none of the statements is correct, you're right! Each of these is an untrue myth. To learn more about staying well hydrated, read below.

We all tend to drink too little water and stay somewhat dehydrated. Did you know that you need about ten 8-ounce glasses of water daily during sedentary days and at least fifteen on days with 20 minutes of moderate exercise? That means you need to drink about one cup of water every hour and a half throughout the day. Mild dehydration has been linked to the development of kidney stones, constipation, and exercise-induced asthma

(Manz 2005). Under-hydration also impairs our concentration, alertness, and memory skills (Ritz 2005).

Your doctor can measure your hydration status with sophisticated blood and urine tests. You can make sure you're getting enough to drink by watching how much you drink and watching your urine color. Believe it or not, looking at the color of your urine is as effective an indicator for your level of hydration as laboratory tests (Kavouras 2002). When you're hydrated, your urine should be straw colored. If you drink a lot of liquids, your urine will become lighter in color. Conversely, if you're dehydrated, your urine will appear darker.

Stay hydrated:

- Always have fresh water for you and your dog
- Refrigerate water bottles or pitchers of water with lemon or lime slices
- Drink 8-10 cups of water each day
- Check your urine for a good straw color
- Drink extra water after exercising
- If you need food after exercising, choose juicy fruits or vegetables

SHOP LIKE A DOG

When I go to the grocery store, I try to stick to my list, but I've drawn to the colorful packages, sample tables, and mega-sized boxes. Before I know it, a few things for dinner becomes a full cart of food I really don't need. Renee W., Cincinnati, OH

We've all gone to the grocery store for a gallon of milk, only to leave with several hundred dollars worth of food and snacks we didn't really need. (Often forgetting to buy the milk that brought us to the store!) Did you ever notice that shopping carts seem to be getting bigger and bigger? And when you go to a warehouse store, you'll probably receive a cart that's big enough for the whole family to sit in! How about the carts at pet stores? That's right—there usually are no carts. Large pet stores may have carts, but they are very small. You come in for a bag of dog food and bottle of shampoo, and that's all you can leave with. You could probably learn a lot about shopping from your dog.

When you enter a grocery store, you're surrounded by glamorous displays and packaging, fun music, and loads of easy-to-reach high-calorie items. There are sections for each of the major food groups—fruits, vegetables, dairy, meats, and breads—but over half of the store may be devoted to snack items—sugary drinks, chips, cakes, cookies, and candies. Go to the pet store and check out your dog's food aisles. There are aisles for "food," stacked with cans and bags of daily nutrition food. And then there are a couple "treat" aisles. One contains "training treats"—these are the treats used to help facilitate your dog's obedience training. These treat bags often suggest using them to reward your dog for following specific commands. There are no instructions to give extra treats to your dog because he's had a bad day, is feeling stress, or is being a good friend in your time of need. The treats are used to reinforce some important behavior. No treats for simply breathing! The other "treat" aisle contains play toys, like balls, Frisbees, and tugging ropes. Comfort toys are also in this "treat" aisle, like chew toys and stuffed animals. There are no sugary sweet or fatty snacks among these treats. Our dogs clearly understand that food is for providing daily nutrition—not a substitute for activity or solution to stress. Small, smelly snacks that make your dog drool are sold in tiny packages, with the understanding that they are the rare treat for doing something really special—not for every day routines. When the dog needs to unwind or relieve some stress, he turns to the toy and comfort aisle—using exercise as a stress reliever rather than sugary, fatty foods. So the next time you're in the supermarket, visit the basic food group aisles for your daily food, get small amounts of snacks for occasional special treats, and get a new toy to encourage you to be more active or a fluffy pillow to use when you need to relax and unwind.

EAT LIKE A DOG RECIPES FOR YOU AND YOUR CANINE FRIEND

When you select a food for your dog, you focus on nutrient-rich foods, high in whole grains, protein, and vitamins. Make these same kinds of selections for yourself. Below are several "dog-approved" recipes for you and your furry friend.

Take these quizzes to see if you know which foods can help your health:
Which 3 foods can help lower your cholesterol:
- ☐ Eggs
- ☐ Almonds
- ☐ Cranberry juice
- ☐ Walnuts
- ☐ Garlic

Which fruits may reduce the effects of aging:
- ☐ Apples
- ☐ Bananas
- ☐ Blueberries
- ☐ Cranberries

Which vegetable may reduce your risk for developing cancer:
- ☐ Corn
- ☐ Onions
- ☐ Radishes
- ☐ Carrots
- ☐ Cucumbers

Read the recipes below to find the answers to these questions.

RECIPES FOR YOU:

Breakfast

High-protein breakfast grill

- **Ingredients**
    - 1 tablespoon of sliced almonds
    - ½ cup of egg substitute or 3 egg whites
    - 2 teaspoons of feta cheese crumbles
    - Ground pepper
- **Preparation**
    - Spray omelet pan with non-stick cooking spray, preferably one made with olive oil.
    - Roast almonds in pan for a couple of minutes, until golden brown.
    - Add egg substitute or egg whites and stir while the egg

cooks.
- Once the egg has cooked and set, sprinkle with feta cheese crumbles. Remove from burner and cover with a lid for 30 seconds.
- Turn onto plate and flavor with ground black pepper.

- **Serving suggestion**
  - Serve with a glass of lemon water and dish of blueberries.
- **Health benefits**
  - **Almonds**

    Almonds are an excellent source of vitamin E, an important antioxidant that acts as a blocker against heart disease. One ounce of almonds supplies almost 7.5 mg of vitamin E. About 24 almonds equals one ounce. The Harvard School of Public Health recommends eating 15 mg of vitamin E daily from foods to get heart protection (http://www.hsph.harvard.edu/nutritionsource/vitamins.html. Accessed September 2008.) You can get this amount by eating just 2 ounces of almonds daily! Other good sources of vitamin E are sunflowers, wheat germ, green vegetables, and tomato sauce. Almonds can also provide a tool for helping to lower cholesterol. Researchers at California State University measured cholesterol levels in people who were fed three diets: a no-almond diet, a low-almond diet (about 1 ounce daily) and a high-almond diet (about 2 ounces daily) (Jambazian 2005). Almond eaters had significantly lower levels of total cholesterol and low-density lipoprotein (LDL) cholesterol (that's the "bad" cholesterol), compared with people not eating almonds. Cholesterol levels dropped in high-almond eaters by 4.5 percent for total cholesterol and 7 percent for LDL cholesterol.

  - **Blueberries**

    Blueberries contain an especially high concentration of antioxidants, which may reduce the risk of developing heart disease and cancer. Blueberries may also reduce aging effects. Studies in aging rats show improvements in memory and learning when rats are fed diets rich in blueberries (Andres-Lacueva 2005). Blueberries may have

other positive effects on slowing aging. When nematode worms were treated with blueberry extracts, their lifespan increased by up to 37 percent (Wilson 2006). Another interesting experiment in rats showed reduced effects of strokes in those rats fed a diet rich in blueberries for one month before their stroke (Wang 2005). Similar studies testing people eating blueberries are needed before we will know whether blueberry-rich diets will similarly slow the aging process in humans.

Cranberry-walnut spread

- **Ingredients**
  - 1 cup fresh apple cider
  - 1 cup sugar
  - ¼ teaspoon cinnamon
  - 1/8 teaspoon nutmeg
  - 12-ounces fresh cranberries
  - ¾ cup pecans chopped
- **Preparation**
  - Heat cider, sugar, and spices in small saucepan until sugar dissolves.
  - Add cranberries and boil until cranberries pop—about 4-5 minutes.
  - Reduce heat and simmer for 30 minutes.
  - Remove from heat. Stir in pecans.
  - Spoon into clean jar and chill in refrigerator. You can also can this in small jars for gifts.
- **Serving suggestion**
  - Serve on your favorite wheat toast or English muffin.
- **Health benefits**
  - **Cranberries**
    Most people know that drinking cranberry juice helps your urinary system and reduces your risk for developing urinary tract infections. Cranberries are also rich in antioxidants that may reduce the risk for heart disease and some cancers. Several experimental studies have shown promise for cranberry consumption decreasing the risk of heart disease and cancer in laboratory studies in animals. A recent study in adults drinking 1½ pints of cranberry juice everyday for 2 weeks, however, showed no improvement in

cholesterol (Duthie 2006). So more studies are needed in humans before we will know if there are more than urinary benefits from cranberries and cranberry juice.
- **Walnuts**
Walnuts are a good source of protein, fiber, B vitamins, and vitamin E. Walnuts are also a great source of omega 3 fatty acids, which have been shown to reduce low-density lipoprotein (LDL) cholesterol—the bad cholesterol associated with heart disease. Many studies have confirmed that eating nuts reduces your risk of heart disease. Researchers at the School of Public Health at Loma Linda University in California reviewed the many available studies (Kelly 2006). They determined that your risk of dying from heart disease decreases by 8 percent for every 30 gram serving of nuts (about ⅓ cup) eaten weekly. So live longer—add walnuts to your breads, salads, cereals, and snacks.

Feather-light nutty waffles

- **Ingredients**
    - 1 cup milk
    - 1 Tablespoon white vinegar or lemon juice
    - ¼ cup egg substitute or one large egg
    - 1/8 cup olive oil
    - 1 cup unsifted flour
    - 2 teaspoons baking powder
    - 1 Tablespoon sugar
    - ¼ cup finely chopped walnuts
- **Preparation**
    - Add vinegar or lemon juice to milk. Let sit for 15 minutes to allow milk to "sour." This will make the waffles extra fluffy.
    - In a separate bowl, mix flour, baking powder, and sugar.
    - Heat waffle iron. I prefer a Belgian waffle maker for this recipe.
    - After milk has soured, add egg and oil and whisk together.
    - Once waffle iron is heated, add liquid to dry

ingredients and gently stir until just mixed. Do not over beat.
- Mix in nuts.
- Cook in waffle iron until golden brown.

- **Serving suggestion**
  - Makes eight 4-inch waffles
  - Serve with real maple syrup, fresh fruit, or cranberry spread (above).
- **Health benefits**
  - This recipe also incorporates the health benefits of **walnuts**. You can also add ¼ to ½ cup of chopped walnuts to your favorite ready-made pancake or waffle mix when you're in a rush to add the goodness of walnuts to your breakfast or brunch.
  - **Maple syrup**
    - Although the amount of calories are the same in real maple syrup and maple-flavored corn syrup, real maple syrup also contains important minerals, like calcium, potassium, and magnesium, that help regulate normal function of the body's cells, bones, muscles, and nerves. Maple syrup also contains small amounts of B-vitamins, including niacin, riboflavin, and pantothenic acid.

Lunch

High-protein lunch grill

- **Ingredients**
  - ¼ cup of egg substitute or 1 egg, scrambled
  - 1 slice of low-fat cheese
  - 2 slices multigrain bread
- **Preparation**
  - Spray one side or each bread slice with non-stick cooking spray, preferably one made with olive oil. Place one slice, coated side down on grill. Place slice of cheese on bread.
  - Spray omelet pan with non-stick cooking spray, preferably one made with olive oil. Heat burner to high heat and pour egg batter into pan. Cook on

one side, moving cooked egg to the center to allow uncooked egg to pour to the edges. When one side is cooked, flip and cook other side. When egg is cooked on both sides, transfer cooked egg to top of cheese.
    - If desired, sprinkle Tabasco sauce on egg.
    - Place second slice of bread over egg, coated side of bread on the outside.
    - Turn on grill and toast sandwich on both sides.
- **Health benefits**
  - **Eggs**
    Eggs are an excellent source of protein, B vitamins, and minerals, including iron and folate. Using only egg whites or an egg substitute gives you the good egg protein without so much cholesterol.

Dinner

Chicken Cacciatore

- **Ingredients**
    - 2 Tablespoons olive oil
    - 4 chicken breasts, rinsed
    - 1 clove garlic, minced
    - 1 medium white onion, chopped
    - 1 medium green pepper, chopped
    - one 14.5-ounce can diced tomatoes
    - one 6-ounce can tomato paste
    - 1 cup white zinfandel or white wine
    - 1 Tablespoon dried parsley flakes
    - ½ teaspoon dried oregano
    - ½ teaspoon dried basil
    - 1 teaspoon sugar
- **Preparation**
    - Heat oil in skillet.
    - Brown chicken breasts in hot oil. Remove chicken and place into 9 x 13 inch baking dish that has been sprayed with vegetable oil spray.
    - Add garlic, onion, and green pepper to skillet. Sauté for 2 minutes, until onions are translucent.
    - Mix remaining ingredients in large bowl. Add garlic,

onion, and pepper mixture. Pour over chicken breasts.
- Bake in 350 degree oven for 45 minutes or until chicken is cooked through. Cooking time may vary, depending on thickness of chicken.

- **Serving suggestions**
    - Serve over cooked fettuccine noodles.
    - Add a green leafy salad as a side dish.
- **Health benefits**
    - **Garlic**
    Garlic has been linked to several health effects. Eating one-half to one clove daily has been shown to reduce cholesterol levels by up to 9 percent (Tapsell 2006). Garlic may also reduce vascular disease by reducing the risk of blood clots and modestly reducing blood pressure (Tapsell 2006).
    - **Tomatoes**
    Tomatoes are rich in lycopene, an important antioxidant linked to reduced risk for cancer and heart disease (Basu 2006). Interestingly, you'll get stronger protection from your heart by eating tomatoes compared with taking supplements rich in lycopene (Das 2006). Tomato juice, tomato sauce, tomato paste, tomato puree, and even ketchup are great sources of lycopene. Cooking tomatoes increases the release of lycopene, so you'll actually get more lycopene from eating cooked tomatoes or tomato products rather than raw tomatoes (Basu 2006). Interestingly, eating tomato products with fats increases the amount of lycopene your body can absorb—so combinations like spaghetti and meatballs, cheese lasagna, and pizza can boost the amount of this important antioxidant (Basu 2006).
    - **Onions**
    Allium plants include onions and herbs, like garlic and chives. In an interesting study in southern Europe, researchers showed that people eating more onions and garlic had a lower risk for developing several types of cancer, including oral and laryngeal cancers, colorectal cancer, breast cancer, and ovarian and prostate cancers (Galeone 2006).
    - **Vegetables**
    Eating vegetables improves your mind. Researchers at Rush University Medical Center in Chicago evaluated cognitive

changes in 3718 adults 65 years old and older and followed for 6 years (Morris, 2006). They found that adults who typically ate more than 2 servings of a vegetable daily had a 40 percent reduction in the amount of mental deterioration over 6 years. This meant their minds looked like they were 5 years younger! All vegetables, except for legumes, slowed loss of intellectual functions. The greatest benefit, however, came from green leafy vegetables.

Waldorf chicken

- **Ingredients**
  - 1/8 cup olive oil
  - 2 Tablespoons butter
  - 2 chicken breasts, sliced into ¼ by ½-1 inch strips
  - 1 large onion, sliced into ¼ inch strips lengthwise
  - 1-2 cloves garlic, minced
  - ½ cup walnut halves
  - 2 gala apples, cored, peeled, and sliced into ½ inch wide sections
- **Preparation**
  - Heat oil and butter in pan on high heat.
  - Add chicken strips and sauté for 15 minutes.
  - Add onion and garlic. Sauté for 5 additional minutes.
  - Add walnuts. Sauté for 5 additional minutes.
  - Add apples. Sauté for 5 additional minutes.
  - Serve with sides of peas and wheat pasta.
- **Health benefits**
  - This recipe also incorporates the health benefits of **walnuts, garlic,** and **onions**.
  - **Apples**

Apples contain a wide variety of phytochemicals that are strong antioxidants. Apples have been linked to reduced risk for cancers, heart disease, asthma, and diabetes (Boyer 2004). Jonagold, red delicious, and Granny Smith varieties are particularly rich in antioxidants (Boyer 2004). Apple peels contain more antioxidants than their flesh, so you can boost the health benefit and add color by leaving on the apple peels.

Citrus spinach salad

- **Ingredients**
  - 3-4 cups fresh baby spinach leaves
  - 1 medium onion, sliced thin
  - 1 11-ounce can mandarin oranges
  - 1/8 cup roasted almond slices
  - Dressing
    - 4 Tablespoons honey
    - 1 Tablespoon olive oil
    - 1 Tablespoon cider vinegar
    - ½ teaspoon cinnamon
    - ½ teaspoon black pepper
    - 1/8 teaspoon salt
- **Preparation**
  - Mix dressing ingredients in a jar and shake vigorously to mix. Refrigerate until ready to use.
  - Make bed of spinach leaves.
  - Arrange onion slices over spinach and top with mandarin orange slices.
  - Sprinkle nuts over salad.
  - Pour dressing over salad immediately before serving and toss gently.
- **Health benefits**
  - Spinach

  Spinach is rich in vitamins, minerals, and fiber. Spinach also contains antioxidants to protect against developing cancer by suppressing tumor growth (Matsubara 2005). For example, prostate cancer cell growth is inhibited with exposure to neoxanthin, a carotenoid antioxidant found in spinach (Kotake-Nara 2001). A diet rich in spinach may help reduce the risk for developing prostate cancer. Spinach consumption has also been linked to a reduced risk of gallbladder cancer. In one study, people who rarely ate spinach had twice the risk of developing gallbladder cancer compared with people eating spinach 3 or more days per week (Rai 2006).

  - Mandarin oranges

  Citrus fruits are rich in vitamins, minerals, and antioxidants. High citrus fruit consumption has been linked to reduced risk for heart disease and cancer. Japanese researchers presented important

information about the health benefits of eating mandarin oranges at the 232nd national meeting of the American Chemical Socity, held in September of 2006. Dr. Sugiura and colleagues found reduced risk for liver disease, atherosclerosis, and insulin resistance (a risk factor for developing diabetes) among people regularly eating mandarin oranges.

Simple green salad

- Make a colorful, nutritious, easy salad that combines the goodness of greens, walnuts, and cranberries.
- Start with a plate of dark green lettuce and fresh spinach leaves.
- Sprinkle with feta cheese.
- Toss on a handful of chopped walnuts.
- Add a handful of dried cranberries.
- Sprinkle with lemon juice or olive oil with vinegar.

Bread-machine cranberry-walnut-wheat bread

- This recipe is designed for a bread machine. Fresh bread is delicious, but devoting a day to kneading, waiting for rising, kneading, etc. is too time consuming. Fluffy would rather have you spend a day jogging with her in the park while the bread machine works its magic at home!
- **Ingredients**
  - ¾ cup plus 2 Tablespoons of low fat or skim milk
  - 2½ Tablespoons of brown sugar
  - 2 Tablespoons of butter
  - 1 cup whole wheat flour
  - 1 cup white flour
  - 1 teaspoon salt
  - 1 teaspoon cinnamon
  - 2 teaspoons active dry yeast
  - ½ cup dried cranberries
  - ½ cup chopped walnuts
- **Preparation**
  - Add milk to the bread machine, followed by the next 6 ingredients.
  - Make a small depression in the flour mixture and add yeast.
  - Allow bread machine to begin mixing dough.

Once ingredients have been mixed together, add in cranberries and walnuts.
- Allow bread machine to continue to mix and process dough. Continue through your bread machine's baking cycle.

Dessert

Peanut biscuits for you

- Preheat oven to 350 degrees
- **Ingredients**
  - 1 cup wheat flour
  - 3 cups rolled oats
  - 1 cup coconut
  - ½ cup butter, softened
  - ½ cup peanut butter
  - 1 cup brown sugar
  - 1 teaspoon vanilla
  - ¼ cup egg substitute or one egg
  - 1/8 cup low fat milk
  - 1 cup unsalted peanuts
- **Preparation**
  - Mix first three ingredients and set aside.
  - Blend butter, peanut butter, and sugar with mixer.
  - With mixer on, add vanilla, egg substitute, and milk.
  - Add first three ingredients to mix. Stir with large spoon until blended.
  - Add peanuts.
  - Scoop out batter with small ice cream scooper. Place on tray sprayed with non-stick spray.
  - Bake for 12 minutes or until cookie is set.
- **Serving suggestion**
  - Serve with low fat milk or low fat yogurt.
- **Health benefits**
  - **Nuts and peanut butter**
    Nuts and nut butters provide a healthy protein source that is naturally rich in healthy unsaturated fats. Eating foods high in unsaturated fats reduces your risk for high

cholesterol, heart disease, and diabetes. Your risk of heart disease decreases by almost 40 percent when you eat nuts four times weekly compared with seldom or never eating nuts (Kelly 2006). This means that you can reduce your heart disease risk by about 8 percent for every serving of nuts you have each week. In addition, the *Journal of the American Medical Association* reported that women who regularly ate nuts and peanut butter had a lower risk for developing adult-onset diabetes (Jiang 2002). Eating peanut butter or one ounce of nuts five or more days per week reduced the likelihood that these women would develop diabetes by 25 percent.

- **Oats**

Oats are a great source of fiber. Diets rich in fiber have been linked to reductions in low-density lipoprotein (LDL) cholesterol (the bad cholesterol) and risk of colon cancer. In one study, men were fed high-fiber cookies every day for 8 weeks (Romero 1998). Those eating cookies with oat bran experienced a 14 percent drop in total cholesterol, 26 percent drop in their levels of LDL cholesterol, and a 16 percent increase in high-density lipoprotein (HDL—the good cholesterol). Triglycerides are another important blood fat that is linked to heart disease. Eating oat bran cookies did not change triglyceride levels in men whose cholesterol was normal; however, triglycerides did drop substantially in patients with elevated levels at the beginning of the study. Among men who had high cholesterol levels before the study started, triglycerides decreased by 28 percent after eating oat bran cookies.

Recipes for MOLLIE

Everyday biscuits

- Preheat oven to 350 degrees
- **Ingredients**
    - 2 cups whole wheat or oat flour
    - ¼ cup milk
    - ¼ cup olive oil
    - ¼ cup egg substitute

- 1 teaspoon garlic powder (optional)
- **Preparation**
    - Mix all ingredients together.
    - Roll onto wax paper to about ¼ inch thickness.
    - Cut small shapes with cookie cutters.
    - Spray cooking sheet with non-stick spray.
    - Bake for 15 minutes. Turn off oven and leave in oven to harden.
    - Store in air tight container or plastic bag.

Peanut butter biscuits

- **Ingredients**
    - 2 cups whole wheat or oat flour
    - 2 tablespoons peanut butter
    - ¼ cup olive oil
    - ¼ cup egg substitute
- **Prepare the same as Everyday Biscuits**

Cheese biscuits

- **Ingredients**
    - 2 cups whole wheat or oat flour
    - ¼ cup grated or shredded cheddar cheese
    - ¼ cup olive oil
    - ¼ cup egg substitute
- **Prepare the same as Everyday Biscuits**

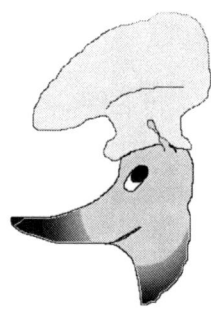

Chapter 3.

Play Like a Dog

> When I was in high school and college, I ran on the cross country and track teams. I was really in great shape. Now after running around after the twins every day, I have no time or interest in doing any exercise. I get enough exercise—I need rest! Michelle V., Ann Arbor, MI

Doctors recommend that adults participate in moderate intensity exercise for 30 minutes most days per week. Unfortunately, less than half of us in the United States actually do this (Macera 2005). One in every five adults does *no* moderate-intensity leisure activity during a typical week (Macera 2005). We've truly become a nation of couch potatoes!

In 2008, the US Department of Labor reported that only 16 percent of Americans 15 years or older participate in exercise on an average day (http://www.bls.gov; accessed September 2008). That's less than one in every five people! The average person reported about 5.1 hours of leisure time every day. The amount of time people spent on an average day exercising was only 17 minutes, compared with 156 minutes or 2.6 hours watching television!

Teenagers spent about 40 minutes exercising and 2 hours watching television daily, while seniors spent only 12 minutes exercising and over 4 hours watching television.

Physical activity has been consistently linked to better overall health. In a recent review of medical research by Dr. Joanna Kruk, the risk of developing a variety of serious health problems was reduced by physical activity and exercise (Kruk 2007):

- Breast cancer risk reduced by 75 percent
- Heart disease risk decreased by 49 percent
- Diabetes risk lowered by 35 percent
- Colon cancer risk decreased by 22 percent

Physical activity also improves our mental health. Researchers at the University of Queensland showed that exercising at least 60 minutes per week resulted in a 30-40 percent reduced risk for having emotional distress and depression (Brown 2005).

Among those who do exercise, walking briskly is the most popular type of moderate exercise. The Centers for Disease Control and Prevention (CDC) recently recommended dog walking to improve the physical activity levels of our society (Ham 2006). For many people who want to exercise, they're not sure how to get started, how much exercise they should really do, how to fit exercise into an already tight schedule, and whether it's all really worth the extra effort anyway. There's so much mis-information people hear about exercise, it's easy to get discouraged. Take the following quiz to see if you can spot common exercise myths.

Choose each statement about exercise that is FALSE:
- ☐ You need to get a least one 30-minute exercise session each day.
- ☐ Exercising less than 30 minutes at a time won't improve your health.
- ☐ You need to sweat to make sure you're exercising hard enough.
- ☐ Don't include your dog in exercise since this will slow you down and reduce your cardiovascular workout.

If you chose every statement as incorrect, you're right on target! (Especially that last one—imagine not wanting to include Precious in your daily exercise!!!) Although we need to get about 30 minutes of exercise each day, we don't have to do all of our exercise in one session. Short exercise periods scattered throughout the day improve your health and fitness level. You can also get good health benefits from a brisk walk—you don't need to be doing a sweat-pouring workout in the gym. Medical research shows that consistent walking is better for your health than infrequent strenuous exercise (Nakamura 2006)—so grab your sneakers, leash, and dog and get started on the road to better health.

LET SAMMY BE YOUR TRAINER

If walking and exercise are so good for us, how come so few of us can stick with a simple exercise program? Dana D., Pittsburgh, PA

This question was asked to about 100 women who had been sedentary before enrolling in a research study (Nies 2006). During the study, they were asked to walk about 90 minutes per week. Even though the vast majority of women noted improvements in physical fitness, overall well-being, and reduced stress, most also reported barriers to maintaining this program. The most common barrier was being too busy and not being able to fit the exercise into a daily routine. Having social support helped maintain the exercise routine for three-quarters of the women. Unfortunately, most of us have days that are already over-scheduled. When we start walking with a friend, an appointment, a cold, or bad weather usually strikes and interrupts the regular exercise schedule. Once you've taken off one day, it's easy to take off two days, and then a week, and then drop exercising all together. This is where turning to your four-legged buddy can be a plus—he's never too busy and can't imagine any reason to skip a day of exercise.

My friend told me it was better to walk without my dog, since Lucky likes to stop to sniff and mark every twig. John U., Upper St. Clair, PA

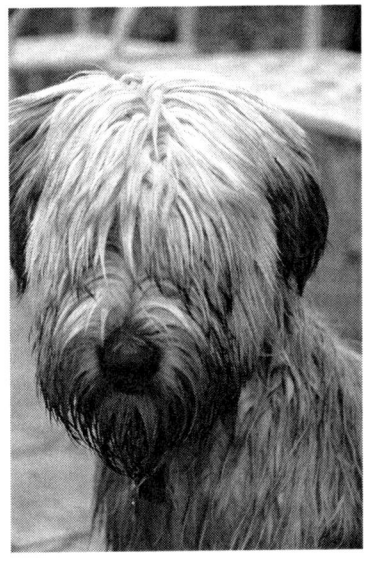

I sure hope Lucky had his ears covered, so he couldn't hear this offensive suggestion!

Even a "bad hair day" won't keep Wheatie from his daily walks.

Yes, Lucky may have you stop a few extra times, but he'll more than compensate for that by using those pleading brown eyes to drag you out to the park each day—rain or shine.

This is a quiz you can take with Lucky. Check off reasons that your dog would prefer NOT to go for a walk:
- ☐ Laundry is piled up.
- ☐ Shopping needs to be done.
- ☐ He went for a walk yesterday.
- ☐ It's raining or might rain.
- ☐ It's cold outside.
- ☐ There's an interesting program on television.

Now don't even try to tell me Lucky picked any of those! Unlike their owners, dogs seem to have an inborn knowledge about the benefits of bounding through the woods or strolling around the neighborhood. For Duke—this is a top priority each day. The good news for you is that Duke's mission is to also make exercise a top priority for you!

A Canadian report showed that dog owners were considerably more physically active than non-owners (Brown 2006). Dog owners walked nearly twice as much as non-owners. An obligation to care for their dogs was frequently cited as the motivation that allowed them to achieve this greater level of physical activity. This point was brought home to me during a wintry January with Wheatie. After spending a weekend laid up in bed with an awful upper respiratory virus, I was able to drag myself out of bed Monday morning so I could see a busy office of patients. Able to leave work a bit early, I returned home mid-afternoon, with visions of pillows and flannel pajamas dancing in my head. When I walked into the house and saw my poor little terrier cooped up in his kennel, expecting to go for a walk, I just couldn't mount the stairs to the bedroom. I don't know if it's because of his long hair and appreciation of cooler temperatures, but my terrier considers snow to be one of Nature's greatest treasures. After, in his view, a disappointingly warm and snow-free winter, the temperatures were now subfreezing and the ground was covered with a delightful layer of soft, powdery fluff. His greatest pleasures are sniffing snow, catching snowflakes, eating great mouthfuls of snow, and rolling in the white stuff until his hair is covered with thick snowballs and he looks like a veritable snow monster. I don't know if it was the fresh, crisp air, the exercise, or watching Wheatie reveal in a simple pleasure, but I felt dramatically better after my walk than before. Since then, I never try to use the "I have a bit of a cold" excuse with Wheatie, trading in a box of tissues for a leash and tennis ball. I have yet to be disappointed by not feeling better after the walk.

LET OMEGA SET YOUR EXERCISE PROGRAM

How much exercise do I need to do? Steve N., Wilkinsburg, PA

The amount of exercise that you and your dog need will vary, depending on your current level of activity and fitness, the intensity of your exercise, and your daily schedule. A good gauge is to ask your dog if he's had enough exercise when you're thinking of stopping any exercise. If you walk half a block or do a couple jumping jacks and then sit down, your dog will cock his head and look at you with a smiling face and wagging tail, clearly expecting longer play. No dog would be satisfied with a 5-minute game of fetch, and neither should you.

Less than half of Americans get an adequate amount of exercise to achieve good health benefits (Macera 2005). The estimated total time for dog walking to achieve health benefits is about 45 minutes per day (Warburton 2006). Walking this amount daily will reduce your risk of dying by 20 to 30 percent (Lee 2001, Myers 2004).

The best way to make sure you achieve your daily walking target is to take daily walks with your dog. Even though dog owners have an enthusiastic, live-in exercise trainer, over half of all dog owners never walk their dogs (Bauman 2001)!

How many days a week should you walk?
- ☐ One
- ☐ Two
- ☐ Three
- ☐ Four
- ☐ Every day

If you're not sure about the answer to this one, just ask Buster. He'll be happy to tell you every day is ideal. Walking only 3 days weekly results in only minimal health benefits (Murtaugh 2005). The other benefit to walking every day is that the walking becomes a regular part of your schedule, like brushing your teeth, so it's easier to make sure you follow through.

VARY YOUR WALKS

I've tried walking on a treadmill and it's BORING! And I just can't get excited about taking the same boring walk every day around my neighborhood with Spotty. Joanna K., Clinton, PA

Walking is more fun for your dog and you when it takes place somewhere with interesting sights, sounds, and smells. Walking through a neighborhood or park is much more refreshing than trudging on a treadmill in the basement. Medical research shows greater physical benefits and exercise enjoyment when walking in the park or neighborhood compared with treadmill walking (Marsh 2006). Dogs also promote outdoor walking for seniors. Researchers at Wake Forest University in North Carolina compared responses to two walking programs—one using a treadmill and one walking in a neighborhood, park, or mall. Walking on the treadmill resulted in a slower pace, shorter strides, and a more negative attitude about the exercise. This study proved what anyone who has walked on a treadmill knows—it's tedious and boring! Walking outdoors or even in a mall, however, provides added distractions to keep our attention focused off of ourselves, allowing us to walk more briskly and with greater enthusiasm and pleasure. Your dog will always choose the walk outdoors instead the treadmill, and so should you!

MAKE DOG WALKS AN ADVENTURE

I'm too busy to take a couple of leisure walks each day. So having to walk the dog just adds extra stress to my day. Brett H., Liberty, PA

Dogs just love walking outside. Their enjoyment seems to come not from knowing that they're exercising muscles and joints, but rather that the walk provides an opportunity to explore the world. Like your dog, you too can sniff the air, listen to the birds, and watch graceful squirrels leap among tree branches overhead. Use all of your senses on your walk. Take a good whiff of life!

When you're a dog, there are two kinds of walks—heel walking and loose-leash walking. Heeling is needed on busy city streets and through crowded sidewalks, when the dog needs to ignore distractions and focus on forward movement through a variety of obstacles. And then there are the more pleasurable, loose-leash walks around the neighborhood, in the park, or through the woods. In the human world, we often use the same high-stress behaviors on our destiny-focused city walks between appointments as we use on what should be our leisure walks. When we turn leisure walks into "power walks," they quickly lose their joy and pleasure.

If you watch most people taking a stroll, they often look very intense. They may be mentally planning strategies for the day's over-scheduled activities, checking their watches, answering emails on ever-present Blackberries, or talking too loudly into a cell phone that seems to be permanently implanted into their head like a Borg from *Star Trek*.

The dog's loose-leash walking is quite the opposite. The dog looks totally relaxed—eyes bright, tail wagging, and tongue lolling out of his mouth in what looks like a devilish grin. He's not concentrating on the walk's destination, the next activity on his list, or tomorrow's breakfast. He's enjoying the moment— reveling in the smells of the flowers, taste of a broken stick, flavors of newly mown grass. As he stops to inspect a grasshopper, jumping back in amazement when the insect hops forward, we shake our heads and say, "Come on. It's only a grasshopper." If Fluffy could speak, she might say, "Only a grasshopper?! Why that creature's a marvel! It effortlessly jumps ten times its length in a single bound. Clearly something worthy of great study."

So the next time you're walking, learn from your dog and mimic his behavior with curiosity and enthusiasm for your environment. No, you don't need to mark your territory every few feet, but do notice the new flowers growing in the neighbor's yard, a slight reddish hue to early autumn leaves, or the burning smell of a fireplace to remind you of campfires as a kid. Revel in these senses and enjoy your walk.

Walks can be a great time to take advantage of unscheduled time for your brain. During my neighborhood walks with Wheatie, I began to notice different landscaping schemes, finally deciding my husband was right—that our all-green front yard would benefit from added color. I had a great opportunity to decide which plants offered the best color, the right size for the spaces between my mature shrubs, and the best longevity. In Pittsburgh, it's also important to identify which plants are least likely to be consumed by our voracious and ever-expanding deer population. While many plants claim they are deer resistant, these walks helped me learn which ones truly lasted all summer without being eaten to the nubbins by enthusiastic herds.

Walks can also serve as a great opportunity for playing pirate with garbage treasures. While many folks are shy about wandering by their neighbor's garbage when it's left out the night before pick up, your pooch will happily sniff unfamiliar items, giving you a great chance to find an assortment of useful riches. If you love scouring garage sales, you'll feel like you have one every week! While out on our walks, we've found wonderful chairs, hanging planters, and bundles of small sticks that made ideal fire kindling. Turning your walk into a scavenger hunt really makes the blocks and miles go by quickly.

SCHEDULE WALKING TIME WITH BROWNIE

My schedule's already so busy, I don't know how I can add a walk in everyday. Kyle O., Monroeville, PA

As I said before, if you can't find time to walk your dog—you're too busy and need to change your schedule. Once you start your exercise program, you'll have the most success if you develop a regular exercise schedule. Suggested schedules are shown below:

Schedule for a mother of school-aged children:
- Morning—walk kids to the bus stop with Fluffy. Walk for 15 minutes after the bus leaves.
- Afternoon—walk Fluffy for 10 minutes and then wait at the bus stop to greet the kids.
- Evening—walk Fluffy with husband around the neighborhood for 20 minutes while dinner is heating up.

Schedule for a wife with a home business:
- Lunch time—take Brutus for a 45-minute hike in the park.
- Evening—take Brutus for a 10-minute walk in the evening before bed.

Schedule for the busy executive
- Morning—take Ginger for 25-minute walk in the neighborhood before leaving for work.
- Evening—take Ginger for a 20-minute walk after work to help wind down before dinner.

The schedule that works best for you will depend on your schedule and your temperament. Try to put your dog in charge of the schedule—these are Fido's walks. When you think about daily walks, don't think about them as *your* walks, but as a necessary requirement from Sergeant Fido. It's okay to say, "I *have to* walk the dog now." You may leave the door grumbling, but after 5 minutes of fresh air and brisk walking, you'll probably be surprised to find yourself whistling, smiling, and happily chatting about your problems with the best listener you could find.

After my sister-in-law had 4 boys, finding time for herself became a major challenge, especially taking time for exercise. Although she felt guilty leaving a house full of chores to go to the gym, she felt more guilty about not walking her golden Labrador with those sad brown eyes. Honey won't care that you're walking because you feel you have to. Your heart and lungs won't care that you'd prefer to catch up on other chores. The important thing is the responsibility you have to caring for your four-legged friend will also help you take better care of yourself.

LET RANGER DECIDE IF IT'S A GOOD DAY FOR A WALK

I'd really like to go walking each day, but I just can't. Brianna B., Bradford Woods, PA

People come up with lots of reasons why they can't stick to an exercise program. Check off reasons you've used in the past to see how you compare with others:

- ☐ Too busy with work or chores
- ☐ No convenient place to walk
- ☐ The weather is often bad
- ☐ I got sick
- ☐ I'm feeling too depressed
- ☐ I'm too tired to exercise

Women asked to walk 90 minutes per week commonly reported each of the above excuses as reasons why they weren't able to keep up with the exercise program (Nies 2006). The most common barrier to exercising was being "too busy," which was reported by 90 percent of the women. Bad weather was a limiting factor for 60 percent of women and half of the women said they were too tired to exercise. So if you chose several of these reasons, you're very similar to other people who have trouble sticking to an exercise routine.

In this same study, having a walking partner was a major factor for women who succeeded in achieving their exercise goal (Nies 2006). Three of four women who met their goal cited having social support or a walking partner to help keep them motivated and on target. There's no better exercise companion than your poodle or retriever. Daisy will be loyal to you and your exercise program. She won't let concerns about cool temperatures, a little rain, or a pile of laundry get in the way of maintaining a healthy routine.

TAKE WATER WITH YOU

Sometimes when I walk, I feel kind of lightheaded and get a headache. When I get home, I eat like a horse, which defeats the weight loss I might get from exercising. Karen T., Ohio Township, PA

In general, people don't drink enough. The average person should drink about 10 glasses of water every day when NOT exercising. If you're exercising, you should drink more. Often, that feeling of being starving after exercising and needing to eat, eat, eat is really the body's way of trying to tell you that you're dehydrated and should drink, drink, DRINK!

Before going out for a walk, drink a big glass or bottle of water. During your walk, carry a bottle of water for you and your dog. Outbound Hound™ makes a nifty water bottle carrier that holds a one-liter bottle and has a front pocket that houses a collapsible bowl. This allows you and your dog to share the same water bottle, with you drinking from the bottle and doggie lapping from the bowl.

After your walk, watch your dog. Invariably, he will head to the nearest water dish and take a long gulp. Even after a long walk, he won't look in his food dish; he knows he needs to replace his water loss. You need to do the same. As soon as you're back at the house, take off your shoes and have 8 to 10 ounces of cool water. This will quench your thirst, replace important fluids you lost on your walk, and reduce your urge to have calorie-laden sodas, fruit drinks, or a sugary snack.

MEASURE YOUR PROGRESS IN MINUTES

I can never get a pedometer to work right and it's a nuisance driving through the neighborhood to figure out how many miles I walked. Susan R., Boston, MA

In order to make a walking program work, it needs to be simple. Trying to measure steps with a pedometer or miles adds enough complexity to make some of us just throw in the towel and forget the whole thing. It's simpler measuring your walks in minutes. It's easier to judge that you can get up 10 minutes early to take the dog out for a 10-minute neighborhood walk before work than figuring out if you have time for a half-mile walk. If your dog is taking extra sniff breaks, you can use a watch to time 5 minutes from the house and then turn around to return home by 10 minutes.

Keep track of your walking progress by using stickers. Place stickers on your refrigerator calendar each time you complete a walk. Count the stickers at the end of the week to make sure you're reaching your walking target. For example, to achieve the healthy target of walking 150 minutes per week, make each sticker count for ten minutes. Every time you walk ten minutes, put a sticker on that date on the calendar. If you walk for 10 minutes in the morning and 20 minutes in the afternoon, you'll place one sticker on the calendar in the morning and two in the afternoon. If you reach your target of thirty minutes per day for five days a week, you'll have three stickers placed on five different days. (Wheatie recommends using bone stickers, but any dog sticker will work fine!) You can also copy and use the *Fit As Fido* monthly walking calendar provided in this book. (See Chart).

Fit As Fido monthly walking calendar

Sunday	Monday	Tuesday	Wednesday	Thursday	Friday	Saturday	Week Total
☐ Fit As Fido ☐ Fit As Fido ☐ Fit As Fido	☐ Fit As Fido ☐ Fit As Fido ☐ Fit As Fido	☐ Fit As Fido ☐ Fit As Fido ☐ Fit As Fido	☐ Fit As Fido ☐ Fit As Fido ☐ Fit As Fido	☐ Fit As Fido ☐ Fit As Fido ☐ Fit As Fido	☐ Fit As Fido ☐ Fit As Fido ☐ Fit As Fido	☐ Fit As Fido ☐ Fit As Fido ☐ Fit As Fido	
☐ Fit As Fido ☐ Fit As Fido ☐ Fit As Fido	☐ Fit As Fido ☐ Fit As Fido ☐ Fit As Fido	☐ Fit As Fido ☐ Fit As Fido ☐ Fit As Fido	☐ Fit As Fido ☐ Fit As Fido ☐ Fit As Fido	☐ Fit As Fido ☐ Fit As Fido ☐ Fit As Fido	☐ Fit As Fido ☐ Fit As Fido ☐ Fit As Fido	☐ Fit As Fido ☐ Fit As Fido ☐ Fit As Fido	
☐ Fit As Fido ☐ Fit As Fido ☐ Fit As Fido	☐ Fit As Fido ☐ Fit As Fido ☐ Fit As Fido	☐ Fit As Fido ☐ Fit As Fido ☐ Fit As Fido	☐ Fit As Fido ☐ Fit As Fido ☐ Fit As Fido	☐ Fit As Fido ☐ Fit As Fido ☐ Fit As Fido	☐ Fit As Fido ☐ Fit As Fido ☐ Fit As Fido	☐ Fit As Fido ☐ Fit As Fido ☐ Fit As Fido	
☐ Fit As Fido ☐ Fit As Fido ☐ Fit As Fido	☐ Fit As Fido ☐ Fit As Fido ☐ Fit As Fido	☐ Fit As Fido ☐ Fit As Fido ☐ Fit As Fido	☐ Fit As Fido ☐ Fit As Fido ☐ Fit As Fido	☐ Fit As Fido ☐ Fit As Fido ☐ Fit As Fido	☐ Fit As Fido ☐ Fit As Fido ☐ Fit As Fido	☐ Fit As Fido ☐ Fit As Fido ☐ Fit As Fido	

Chart instructions: Check a *Fit As Fido* box every time you walk for 10 minutes. Your target is to walk at least 150 minutes per week—so 15 or more boxes should be checked each week. Write your total number of 10-minute walks in the Week Total column. If the number is 15 or more, circle the smiling Fido.

Make sure you vary your walk location to help keep walks interesting for you and your dog. If you usually turn right when you leave the house, try turning left instead. Or try walking on the other side of the street, giving your dog new smells and you new views. Look for nearby areas that provide greater physical challenges, like hills, ruts to jump over, and tree branches to dunk under, to help change the intensity of your outings and engage different muscle groups in exercise.

Change the tempo of your walks. Every walk doesn't need to be at the same pace and don't be afraid to change pace during an individual walk. If you take your dog to a leash-free dog park, you'll notice that he doesn't exercise like a human. Humans will do a short warm-up, then jog or power walk for most of their exercise time, and maybe follow this with a short cool down. Dogs, on the other hand, will do some stretches, warm up with a slow walk, and then intermix bursts of running and slow walking. Try this on your walks with your dog. After walking for a few minutes, ask your dog to hurry up and run alongside you as you jog. A few minutes later, slow back to a walk. Mix in some skipping or jumping along the way. When you come to a curb or crack in the sidewalk, leap over it. Your dog will love it and you'll get better exercise than just walking at the same pace.

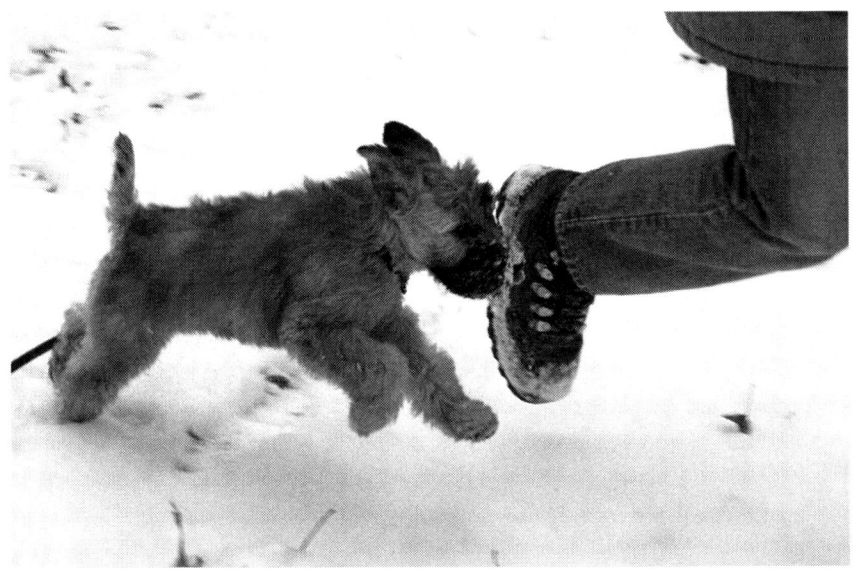

Add short runs and skips to your daily walks to vary the pace, improve your exercise, and keep you and your dog entertained.

KEEP A BASKET OF WALKING SUPPLIES HANDY

I went hiking with my friend and when my dog and I came back, I was wet and muddy and so was she. It took me an hour to get everything cleaned up. Liz G., Mars, PA

When you decide to make walking part of your regular routine, you'll need to have gear set aside and maintained for you and your dog so walking is easy in all weather. Here's a list of items you'll need:
- Six foot leather leash
- Water bottle
- Dog poopie bags
- Training treats

- Rain gear and umbrella
- Walking shoes and boots
- Dog comb and brush to brush out twigs and leaves
- Consider having a filled watering bucket and towel outside your door to wash off Toby's muddy paws before re-entering the house.

To make walking easy, have everything together in an easy-to-store-and-reach spot. I keep everything for the dog in a basket by the back door. If you're planning long walks, make sure you take a bottle of water—for you and Buddy. Take a small, collapsible water dish along for Buddy. That way, you can pour water in the bowl for Buddy, and still have a bottle that hasn't been slobbered for you to drink. I also bought a small purse that can hold my driver's license and credit cards, some cash, a few dog treats, the collapsible water dish, and about six poopie bags. After a few months, I added a little poopie bag dispenser on a chain to my purse. It holds 15-20 disposable bags, so I'm always prepared. The little bag dispenser is a great reminder to walk the dog and a great conversation starter! These supplies are in my everyday purse. So if I'm walking in the neighborhood, park, or pet store, I always have all of my essentials with me and no excuse not to take Wheatie along. If you prefer to use a bigger purse for everyday, just slip the little dog purse inside. It will remind you to take a walk when you're reaching inside to get your wallet to stop at the ice cream booth for a double-scoop sundae.

STOCK UP ON ALL-WEATHER WALKING GEAR

It's too much work to walk when it's bad weather. I have to get myself all bundled up and then clean River's muddy feet before we can go back in the house. Debbie R., Fox Chapel, PA

Make sure your hall closet is stocked with good walking gear for you. Proper clothing is also a must. Your dog won't care if you have designer labels on your clothes or the latest athletic wear. You *do* need to make sure you have supportive walking shoes and hiking boots for mud, rain, and snow. (Yes—your dog *will* still want to walk in all kinds of weather!) If you keep your feet dry in boots, and use a rain coat and umbrella, walking in the rain should not be a problem. If you don't want your dog to get wet and dirty, keep him on a neighborhood or park path instead of a wooded hike on rainy days.

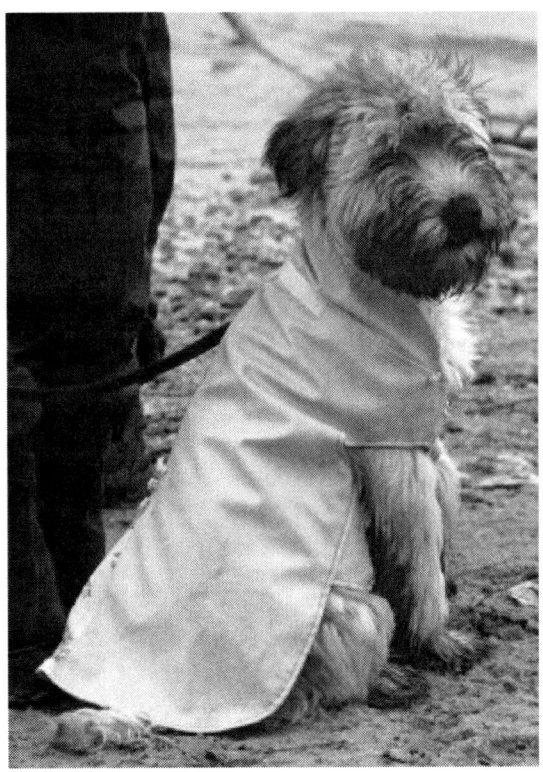

Be prepared for any kind of weather. Don't let a bad forecast dampen your motivation for exercise and play. (Photo courtesy of Julie Milone.)

If you do hike in the woods, and both your dog and I would recommend that you do, remember he's likely to pick up leaf pieces, seeds, twigs, and sometimes burrs. My long-haired dog used to hate being groomed until we incorporated a quick grooming session into our walks. When we return home, Wheatie is not allowed back in the house until he's been quickly brushed. He stands on a bench by the back door, while I go through his hair with a brush and comb. If you have a long-haired dog like I do, keep a bottle of spray conditioner, a slicker brush, and a de-matting brush in your grooming basket. Spray Lady down with conditioner before starting to brush. Brushing will also remove loose dirty, so she'll be beautiful and fluffy once she dries. I also keep a plastic garden watering can by the back door. Before Wheatie comes in, I "water" his muddy feet with the can, which I have found is easier than taking out the hose or putting him in the sink in the house. If Lady still has a bit of that wet dog smell, spray her with a dog deodorant. I like Nova Pearls™ by Tomlyn®. It's unbelievably effective on a smelly dog and leaves your dog smelling fresh and not perfumed.

In the fall, we added a blaze orange vest to Wheatie's small hiking wardrobe. The vest protects him from novice hunters in the woods and makes him more visible to me when doing off-leash hikes. Another advantage is that the vest covers his sides and underbelly, so there are fewer exposed areas to capture mud, twigs, and burrs.

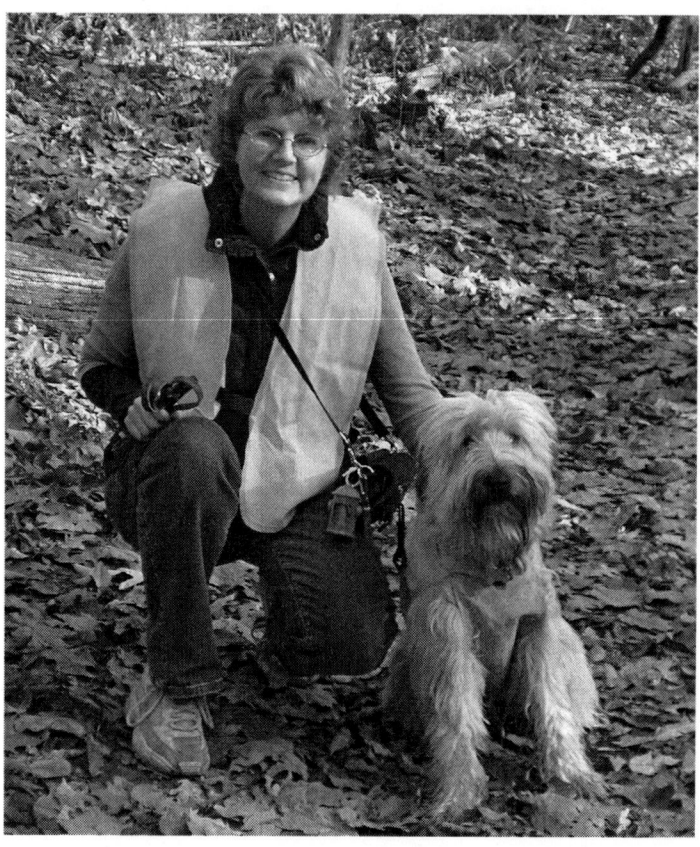

Blaze orange vests provide protection from hunters and burrs.

TAKE THE WHOLE PACK WALKING

I'm happy to take evening walks, but there's no way the rest of family will. I've tried getting my kids and mother-in-law to go walking before.
Georgia T., Plum, PA

When my boys were little, I loved taking them for walks in the neighborhood and the woods. They'd marvel at mom's vast knowledge of nature, like how maple seeds become helicopters or pill bugs turn into tiny balls when scared. Once they hit middle school, they'd rather talk with friends, play computer games, or even do homework than go for a stroll with the old lady. I still doubt they'd come if I asked them to walk with me, but my now-teenagers will usually "come help take Wheatie for a walk." These walks provide good exercise for all of us and a great time to chat about school, friends, and dreams in a low pressure, non-nagging environment.

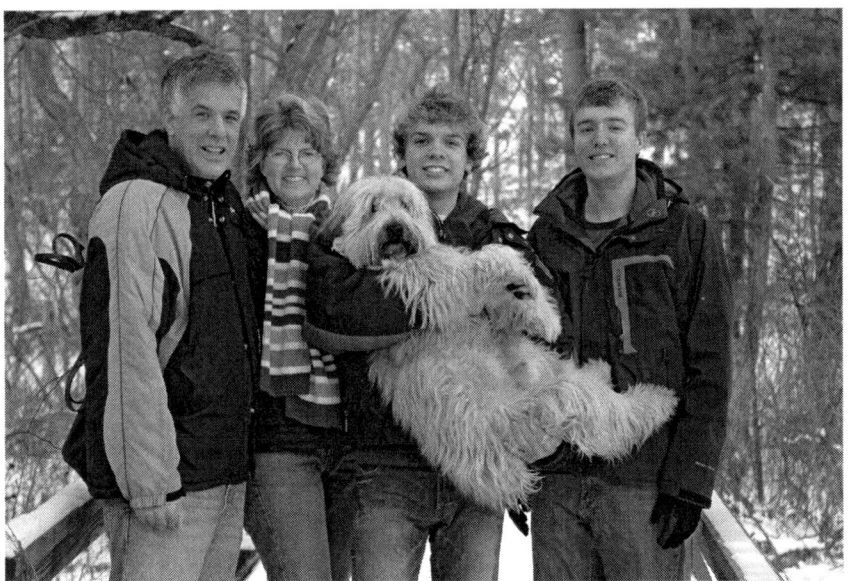

Wheatie helps bring the family together for Sunday hikes in the park.

The same will probably be true with your parents or in-laws. My parents grew up in a time when you worked hard all day to make a living, and people didn't have a lot of leisure time. As working adults, their peers generally didn't plan visits to the gym, workouts with buddies, or weightlifting sessions. Using free time for exercise may seem odd to some seniors. Most seniors, however, are hard workers and miss having daily tasks, like preparing meals for a big family, doing laundry, making lots of beds, or going to work every day. They may welcome an important family chore and will probably be more willing to go to the park if it's to "walk the dog" rather than to "walk Grandma." Remember, walks should be fun for you and your dog. Shout a cheery, "Walk!" and make sure this brings a smile to both your face and your dog's.

Make a walking program work for you:

- Measure your walks in minutes, not miles or steps
- Vary your walk
- Vary your walking speed
- Look for safe routes with hills
- Keep an area of walking gear ready

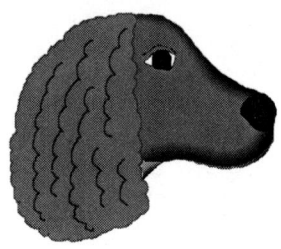

Chapter 4.

Sleep Like a Dog

When I was a kid, I hated naps and early bed times. I used to promise Mom, "When I'm grown-up, I'll never sleep!" I guess I got my wish. Now I'd give anything to get a good night's sleep. How come I can't just plop down like Scruffy and go to sleep? Christie F., Dayton, OH

The expression, "It's a dog's life," conjures up the image of the lazy hound, collapsed in a state of prolonged, blissful sleep on the front porch. Dogs are certainly great sleepers and we can learn a lot about embracing good sleep habits from our dogs. Unfortunately, there are many myths about sleep that encourage us to adopt bad sleeping habits. Take the quiz below to see if you can spot the false sleep myths.

Select each statement about sleep that is NOT correct:
- ☐ If you're having trouble going to sleep, try watching television in bed for 20 minutes.
- ☐ A half glass of wine will relax you before bed and help you get a better night's sleep.

☐ Avoid snacks after dinner. Food eaten before bed doesn't get burned off and turns to fat.
☐ It's okay to sleep just a few hours during the week, as long as you make up the sleep on the weekends.

If you picked every statement as incorrect, you're a smart sleeper. To find out the truth about sleep, read the chapter below.

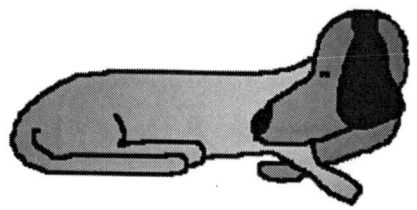

POOR SLEEPERS HAVE LOTS OF COMPANY

As a kid, I hated going to bed. Now that I'm in my forties, I'd love a good night sleep. When I want to sleep, I can't? Do other people have sleep problems like me? Paula E., McKeesport, PA

Poor sleep is very common. The National Sleep Foundation surveys adults in the United States using the Sleep in America poll (National Sleep Foundation 2008). Although the National Sleep Foundation recommends getting 7-9 hours of sleep nightly, the average American in 2008 slept 6 hours and 40 minutes at night on weekdays and 7 hours and 25 minutes at night on the weekends. Interestingly, these same people reported needing to sleep 7 hours and 18 minutes on average to function at their best. Three of every ten people surveyed reported needing at least 8 hours of sleep at night, while only two in ten successfully achieved this target. Americans are sleeping less than they used to. In 1998, one in every three adults reported sleeping 8 or more hours per night on week nights. This dropped down to only one in four adults in 2005. In the 2008 survey, poor sleep was linked to difficulties with daily tasks with poor sleep resulting in work tardiness during the preceding month for one in ten adults and falling asleep or being very sleepy on the job for almost one in three adults. And one in three drivers reported nodding off or at least briefly falling asleep while driving.

Even among people who get a good number of hours of sleep each night, many people feel their sleep is restless, light, or of poor quality. This has been described as *non-restorative sleep*. A survey of 25,580 Europeans from seven countries found that 11 percent reported non-restorative sleep (Ohayon, 2005). People experiencing non-restorative sleep were over twice as likely to report moderate to severe physical and intellectual fatigue. They were over three times more likely to report a moderate to severe decrease in effectiveness, memory problems, and mood problems (including irritability, depression, and anxiety).

LEARN TO RECOGNIZE NORMAL SLEEP

If so many people have problems sleeping, how do I know if I'm getting normal sleep? Lilie H., Lincoln Park, MI

We often think that sleep is the time when the body shuts down, like turning off a switch on a robot. Actually, sleep is a very dynamic process, with lots of brain activity. You sleep in cycles, with each cycle lasting about 90 to 100 minutes. During each cycle, your brain passes through five important stages of sleep: stages 1, 2, 3, and 4 and then dream sleep. Dream sleep is known as rapid eye movement or REM sleep, because your eyes move back and forth during this stage of sleep. Stages 1 and 2 are the lightest stages of sleep. When you take a nap, you're in these light stages and it's easy for someone to quickly wake you up. During Stage 1 sleep, you may have a feeling that you're falling and involuntarily jerk, waking yourself up. (How many times have I done that while sitting in a boring class or riding in the passenger seat of a car before jerking my head up and announcing, "I'm awake!") Stages 3 and 4 are deeper sleep. These are the stages where you need to shake someone to wake him up. When you wake up from stages 3 or 4, you may feel temporarily confused and disoriented for a few minutes. Most of us have had that experience where you're woken up and for a few minutes you're not sure where you are. This happens when you wake up during deep sleep. During REM sleep, your heart beats faster, breathing quickens, and your arms and legs don't move. During REM sleep, you'll have the most vivid dreams. We generally can remember our dreams if we wake up during REM sleep.

RECOGNIZE YOUR SLEEP NEEDS

Since I turned forty, I don't think I'd recognize a good night's sleep. I try to sleep about 6 hours a night, but I don't know if that's enough. Brian N., Clarksburg, WV

Many people wonder if they're getting enough sleep. Take the quiz below to see if you know how much sleep is enough. Pick the correct statement or statements about sleep:

☐ As we get older, we need less and less sleep. So once you're middle-aged, 6 hours a night is enough.
☐ There are no long-term problems from sleeping too little.
☐ People who sleep less can accomplish more by being more productive.
☐ Teenagers who get up at 6 a.m. should be asleep by 9 p.m.

Believe it or not, the only correct statement is that teenagers need early bed times. After you read this chapter, you'll become a sleep expert to help improve your own sleep and the sleep of your family.

Sleep patterns changes with age. Newborn babies generally sleep most of the time. They usually sleep between 8 and 10 hours during the day and another 8 to 10 hours during the night. By 6 months, sleep usually decreases to about 14 hours a day. After reaching age 1 and until school starts, most kids need 10 to 12 hours of sleep each day. Even though they may give up an afternoon nap, preschool-aged kids still need about 10 to 12 hours of sleep a night. Once they start school, most kids need about 10 hours each night. Teenagers still need more than 9 hours of sleep each night. Unfortunately for them and their parents, teens usually have to get up earlier to catch the school bus and prefer to stay up late chatting with friends and watching movies. (You parents of teens—good luck!) Adults need a little less sleep, about 7 to 8 hours each night.

As adults age, there's a common myth that they no longer need much sleep. Older adults still need about 8 hours of sleep, although they may have to adjust their sleeping patterns to get it. Chemicals that regulate sleep (like cortisol, growth hormone, and melatonin) vary with age, causing significant changes in our sleep patterns (Blackman 2000, Cajochen 2006). As we age, we usually begin feeling sleepy earlier and need to take advantage of an earlier bed time to easily get to sleep. By middle age, we should plan an earlier bed time. We will also notice that our sleep will be lighter and we'll wake up more often during the night. Seniors tend to have more episodes of waking up during the night and usually an earlier time when their body feels ready to end the night's sleep. Older folks, therefore, usually have to adjust their sleep habits to avoid getting too little sleep during the night and then feeling excessively sleepy during the day. People who don't adjust their sleep habits often find themselves napping excessively during the day, which can further disrupt good night time sleep.

Nightly sleep requirements at different ages:

- Newborns – 16 to 20 hours
- Toddler – 10 to 12 hours
- Elementary student – 10 hours
- Teenager – more than 9 hours
- Adult – 7 to 8 hours

Not only does the amount of time we snooze change with aging, but our sleep patterns change as well. Newborns spend about half of their sleep time in REM sleep. The next time you see a baby sleeping, look closely. About half of the time, you'll see little eyes moving back and forth under the eyelids, letting you know the wee one is dreaming. As adults, we tend to lose REM sleep. Younger adults spend half of their sleep in the lighter Stage 2 sleep and only 20 percent in REM sleep. As we age, lighter sleep occurs more and REM sleep occurs less and less. This may be part of the reason that older adults will wake up more frequently—they're spending more and more time in lighter stages of sleep that are easier to be aroused out of.

UNDERSTAND THE IMPORTANCE OF A GOOD NIGHT'S SLEEP

But mommy, why do I have to go to bed? Steven M., Atlanta, GA

When my two very active little boys used to ask this question, a very honest answer might have been, "Because your dad and I need some quiet time!" Luckily, however, I knew the better answer, "Because sleep makes you get big and strong." When you're growing, your brain pumps out growth hormone while you sleep. Getting at least 9 hours of sleep each night helps make sure your child's body has enough time to make a good amount of growth hormone. As adults, we no longer need to use sleep for growth. Adequate sleep for adults, however, still has many important health benefits.

My dog sleeps half of his life away. Luckily, I can get by with only about 5 hours of sleep a night. Brian M., New York, NY

Sleep should not be looked at as a luxury. Not only do we feel tired, depressed, and grumpy after a poor night's sleep, but almost 3 in 10 people have missed work, made work errors, or missed other activities because of sleep problems (National Sleep Foundation 2008). If you're not sleeping well, you'll also probably affect your partner's sleep. In their 2005 survey, the National Sleep Foundation found that people lost an average of 49 minutes of sleep at night due to their partner's sleep problem (National Sleep Foundation 2008).

Believe it or not, sleep also has many important general health benefits. Take this quiz to see if you know what benefits you might expect from adopting a healthy sleep pattern. Which of the following health conditions is/are worse when you don't get enough sleep:
- ☐ Obesity
- ☐ Diabetes
- ☐ Heart disease
- ☐ Migraines
- ☐ High blood
- ☐ Infections

If you picked every condition, you're absolutely right! Getting enough sleep makes us feel more energized and improves our attitude. Just like mom used to tell us, sleep is also important for the rest of our body.

A survey of students ages 17 to 30 years old showed that people sleeping only 6 to 7 hours nightly were 50 percent more likely to report having poor health compared with people getting a full night's sleep (Steptoe 2006). Those sleeping less than 6 hours nightly were twice as likely to have poor health. A large survey of over 200 million adults in the United States found that almost one in five had trouble sleeping (Pearson 2006). Those individuals with sleep problems were more likely to have health problems with obesity, high blood pressure, congestive heart failure, anxiety, and depression. So take a lesson from your dog and make sleep a regularly scheduled priority to improve your energy level, your mood, your function, and your health.

SLEEP STRENGTHENS YOUR HEART

Sleep deprivation causes an imbalance in chemicals, such as cortisol, epinephrine, norepinephrine, and magnesium (Takase 2004). These chemicals are important messengers for the autonomic nervous system, which controls automatic body functions like heart beat and breathing. Even in healthy people, an imbalance in these chemicals from sleep deprivation can cause a strain on the heart (Takase 2004). Sleep loss also increases chemicals that cause inflammation, which is another important risk factor for heart disease, as well as arthritis and diabetes (Irwin 2006).

The effects of sleep deprivation on the heart were studied in a group of over 70,000 nurses, who were followed for 10 years (Ayas 2003). Among these women, those sleeping 5 or fewer hours each night had almost twice the risk of experiencing heart disease compared with women sleeping 8 hours at night. Adults who don't get enough sleep are also more likely to have problems with their blood pressure. In a study of 3620 adults between ages 32 and 59 years old, people typically sleeping 5 or fewer hours per night were over twice as likely to have high blood pressure compared with people sleeping 7 to 8 hours per night (Gangwisch 2006).

SLEEP CURBS YOUR APPETITE

Our bodies and those of other animals have developed so that sleep triggers important appetite-suppression mechanisms (Vanitallie 2006). The brain links wakefulness with hunger and food-seeking behavior. So if we're short-changing ourselves on sleep, our bodies will insist that we eat more than we need to. Some people think they eat less when they're sleeping more because they have fewer hours awake when they can overeat. While this is true, it's important to remember that staying up late makes us want to overeat because we lose our body's natural appetite suppressant—sleep!

Since sleep and appetite are linked, it's not surprising that poor sleep has also been linked to obesity. Researchers at Columbia University monitored weight over 10 years in adults in the United States (Gangwisch 2005). People who reported sleeping less than 7 hours per night were more likely to develop obesity compared with people who slept 7 or more hours nightly. The less people slept, the more overweight they were. Excess weight was highest in those people sleeping the fewest hours each night. People sleeping only 2 to 4 hours each night were over twice as likely to be obese as people sleeping 7 hours or more. The risk for being obese was 60 percent higher in people sleeping 5 hours each night and 27 percent higher among those sleeping 6 hours.

SLEEP CONTROLS YOUR BLOOD SUGAR

Your body carefully regulates your blood glucose levels while you sleep, so you don't experience a drop in blood sugar levels even though you've fasted for 7 or 8 hours (Spiegel 2005). If you lay down for 7 or 8 hours, don't eat, and stay awake, your blood sugar levels will drop. While you sleep, your body carefully adjusts sugar levels, changing your metabolism when you're in light and deep stages of sleep. Sleep restriction harms your body's natural ability to properly regulate blood sugar levels (Spiegel 2005). Changes in metabolic hormones in people who have chronic sleep deprivation may result in increased risk for insulin resistance and diabetes.

Researchers in Sweden surveyed a sample of about 1200 adults, asking questions about their health and sleep patterns (Mallon 2005). Twelve years later, they repeated their examinations to determine which people developed diabetes. They found that men sleeping 5 or fewer hours nightly had a nearly 3 times greater risk of developing diabetes. Men reporting difficulty staying asleep were almost 5 times more likely to develop diabetes. Interestingly, women with sleep problems did not have a higher risk for developing diabetes. The researchers noted that, in general, men seem to be more susceptible to general health problems with sleep disturbance than women. A similar study of over 1500 men followed for about 16 years in the United States likewise found that men sleeping 6 or fewer hours nightly were twice as likely to develop diabetes (Yaggi 2006). In their survey, those men with excessive sleep (over 8 hours nightly) also had a higher risk of becoming diabetic.

Among people who have diabetes, sleep deprivation has been linked to poorer blood sugar control (Knutson 2006). Furthermore, diabetics with a higher sleep debt are more likely to have major diabetes complications, such as diseases of the peripheral nerves, retina, kidneys, or heart. So maintaining a good sleep pattern may be an important step to getting and keeping your diabetes under better control.

SLEEP REGULATES YOUR IMMUNE SYSTEM

Your immune system is also regulated by sleep. Sleep regulates several hormones that play important roles in keeping immune factors balanced, including corticotrophin-releasing hormone, growth hormone, cortisol, and prolactin (Bryant 2004, Lange 2006). Levels of immune factors can be negatively affected by sleep deprivation, although the effects seem to vary, based on the amount of sleep deprivation (Bryant 2004). Interference with the normal immune system with poor sleep may increase risk for developing infections and other immune conditions.

SLEEP REDUCES YOUR SENSITIVITY TO PAIN

Most people develop a pain problem at some time. As a matter of fact, a pain complaint is one of the most common reasons for people to see their doctors. For anyone who has developed a pain problem, you'll probably remember having trouble sleeping. Did you also know that not sleeping enough actually lowers your pain threshold? Sleep experts at the Henry Ford Health System conducted pain experiments in healthy adults who did not have any pain complaints (Roehrs 2006). Everyone was tested with the same painful heat—testing how hot the stimulus had to get before it was perceived as painful. Before pain testing, people were assigned to different sleep conditions. People who were allowed to spend 4 hours in bed at night had their pain threshold lowered by one-fourth compared with people who were allowed to spend 8 hours in bed. People who experienced disrupted sleep with no REM or dream sleep had their pain threshold lowered by one-third compared with people who were allowed to experience REM sleep. These experiments show that poor quality or short sleep make you more susceptible to pain—something that doesn't seem painful to the person with normal sleep will seem painful when you haven't slept well. The researchers for this study speculated that if you already have a pain problem—like arthritis, fibromyalgia, or low back pain—having disrupted sleep could actually make that pain worse.

SLEEP IMPROVES MIGRAINES

When the environment gets dark at night, the brain produces an important sleep chemical, called melatonin. Bed time melatonin levels have been checked in people with and without migraine headaches (Claustrat 1989). People with migraines have melatonin levels that are only two-thirds as high as the headache-free folks. This may explain why about one in three people with migraines complain of trouble falling asleep and staying asleep (Kelman 2005).

When people with migraines don't sleep enough, their migraines are more likely to be more frequent and more severe. Migraine sufferers who regularly sleep 6 or less hours at night have over 20 percent fewer headache-free days and almost 25 percent more days with severe headaches (Kelman 2005).

Health problems associated with sleep deprivation

- Heart disease
- High blood pressure
- Obesity
- Diabetes
- Increased infection risk
- Pain
- Migraines

ADD SLEEP TO YOUR SCHEDULE

I don't have the time to sleep away 8 hours at night! Diane T., Fairmont, WV

In today's fast-paced, text-messaging, emailing, get-it-done-yesterday world, our employers, volunteer organizations, and kids often make us wish we had more than 24 hours available in a day. Many people try to cut out sleep to fit too many activities into over-structured and over-committed lives. Take the quiz below to look for the best ways to get by on too little sleep.

If you can't sleep 8 hours at night, what's the best way to keep yourself alert and high-functioning:

☐ Drink coffee
☐ Do jumping jacks or another aerobic exercise for 5 minutes every 30 minutes
☐ Sing or talk out loud
☐ Eat a high carbohydrate meal
☐ Eat a high protein meal

Unfortunately, you can't trade sleep for caffeine, activity, or food. If you can't fit in 8 hours of sleep, you probably need to simplify your schedule, cut down on out-of-the-house or volunteer commitments, and spend a bit more time taking care of yourself and your health.

Strategies to make sure you make time for sleep

- Stick to regular bed times during the week
- Get up early and at the same time each day
- Don't skip breakfast
- Eat at least 2 of your meals each day at the kitchen or dining table
- Choose only one important volunteer activity
- Divide household chores among the family
- Use carpools to help ferry kids
- Prepare several dinner entrees each Monday, so you're ready all week
- Limit caffeine, alcohol, and nicotine
- Talk to one friend for at least 15 minutes every day

DON'T SUBSTITUTE COFFEE OR FOOD FOR SLEEP

As long as I have a pot of coffee going, I can get by with very little sleep. Sue S., Newark Valley, NY

My sister-in-law is a big coffee drinker, with a percolator often going almost around the clock. She gets very little sleep and thinks she's doing fine, as long as she "has her coffee." We all know if we don't get enough sleep, we feel sluggish and less mentally alert. This is a big reason professional drivers, like long-distance truck drivers, need to take a required sleep break. Sleep recharges our mental batteries so we can once again be bright and alert.

Sleep experts in Switzerland found that sleep deprivation temporarily worsened people's mental capabilities (Gottselig 2006). When these same sleep-deprived people had caffeine, simple mental processes did improve. Complex mental activities, however, do not improve with caffeine. So don't use caffeine to avoid feeling the need for sleep. Taking the time to get adequate sleep will improve your performance and productivity, making up for the time "lost" by sleeping.

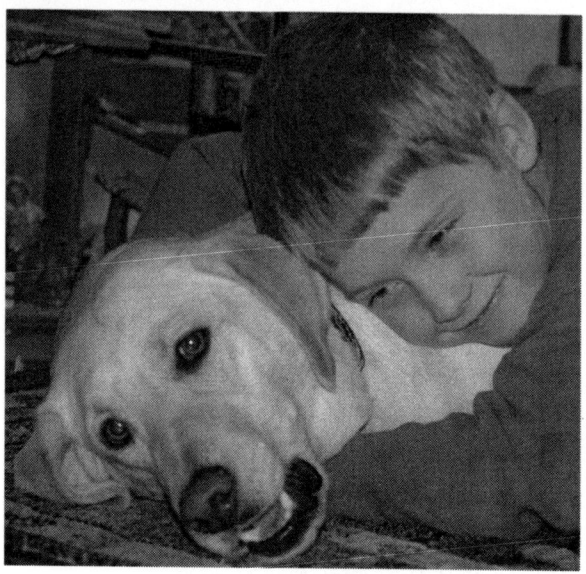

Embrace a good night's sleep

DON'T BE AFRAID TO TAKE A NAP

As soon as the kids get home from school, Pepper retreats to his cage for a nap. Wish I had the luxury of taking naps during the day! Sharon S., Columbus, OH

Pepper has the right idea. Naps can be good for your health—even when you're an adult! The 2008 National Sleep Foundation survey found that 46 percent of people took 2 or more naps during the preceding month, with naps lasting 1 hour on average (National Sleep Foundation 2008). You may be surprised to learn that there has been a lot of medical research looking into napping. (And you thought your doctor was golfing when you couldn't reach him in the afternoon. He may have been studying napping!)

Taking a short mid-afternoon nap can help rejuvenate you for the evening's activities. People who take a short afternoon nap tend to have more energy and are more alert after their nap. Taking short naps has also been linked to a reduced risk for heart attacks (Dhand 2006, Naska 2007). A large survey of almost 24,000 healthy adults evaluated napping habits and the occurrence of heart disease over an average follow-up of almost six and one-half years (Naska 2007). After taking into consideration other risk factors for heart disease, like age, smoking, and obesity, people who regularly napped at least three days per week for at least 30 minutes per nap had a 37 percent decreased of dying from heart disease. Taking several naps a day or spending a long time napping, however, is bad for your health (Dhand 2006).

Researchers have determined that naps give the best health benefits when they are:

- About 30 minutes long
- Taken at around 3:00 in the afternoon
- No more than once a day

If you find that you want to nap for longer than 45 minutes or several times a day, you may be having sleep problems at night and should talk to your doctor.

AVOID CAT NAPS

I'll close my eyes for 10 or 15 minutes in the afternoon for a short cat nap. Is that helpful? Helen T., Morgantown, WV

As you might guess, any dog will tell you that taking "cat" naps can't be good for your health! Once again, Duchess is right—naps need to last about 30 minutes to get good restorative benefits. Researchers at Hiroshima University in Japan found that people felt less tired after taking very short naps, but their performance was worse and they felt more depressed (Hayashi 2005). When people took a naps lasting at least 30 minutes, their performance and mood both improved. These researchers discovered that naps when your body experiences only the lightest sleep (Stage 1) don't give your body the restorative benefits of a longer nap. In order for a nap to be recuperative, you need to have Stages 1 and 2 of sleep, which typically takes about 30 minutes.

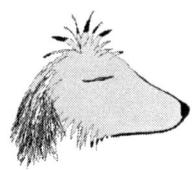

ARRANGE YOUR SLEEP PATTERN

I try to get a good night's sleep, but I toss and turn and worry about what I need to get done. Dolores G., Miami, FL

As parents, we usually implement a regular, predictable bed time routine for our small children who'd rather be racing around the house or for those little puppies we're trying to housebreak. Every parent and puppy owner soon learns that sticking to this routine is comforting for child and dog and promotes more successful falling asleep and sleeping through the night.

- **SET UP A SLEEPING DEN**

Have a designated sleep spot—not in front of television, on the sofa, or in the recliner. Your sleep spot should have only two purposes—sleep and snuggling with and loving your mate. Don't use your bed for anything other than these two important activities. Your bed should not be your place for reading, snacking, or watching television. If you go to bed and can't fall asleep, get out of bed and go to a chair to unwind and read quietly for 15 minutes before returning to bed to sleep. When you get up in the morning, make your bed. A bed that's made looks less accessible for crawling into to read a book or watch a television show than one with unturned cover inviting you in.

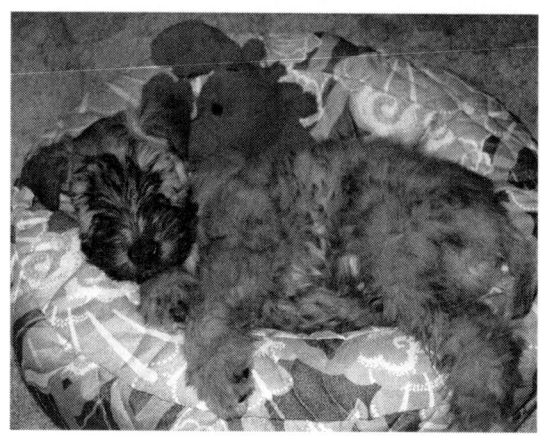

Plan to sleep in your bed—not the sofa, recliner, or television lounge

- **LIMIT CAFFEINE, ALCOHOL, AND NICOTINE**

Both caffeine and alcohol can impair sleep. Caffeine should be avoided in the evening if you have sleep problems. Drinking too much caffeine tends to reduce your total sleep time and makes it more likely that you'll wake up during the night. In general, it's best to limit caffeinated beverages to 2 cups per day. (Remember—most mugs contain 2 cups of liquid.) When calculating your caffeine intake, remember to include caffeinated sodas in addition to coffee and tea. Most hot chocolate has very little caffeine.

Some people like having a cocktail before bed because the alcohol makes them feel drowsy. Although you may feel sleepy after drinking, alcohol often prevents your brain from entering the deeper, more restorative stages of sleep.

Nicotine can also affect sleep. Epidemiologists at Johns Hopkins Medical Center compared sleep patterns in smokers and non-smokers (Zhang 2006). Smokers took longer to fall asleep and experienced less total sleep time than non-smokers. In addition, smokers spent more of their sleep time in the lightest sleep (Stage 1 sleep). These changes in sleep pattern may be an important cause of sleep disturbances among smokers.

- **EXERCISE EACH DAY**

Whether it's our dogs or our kids, we know there will be a good night's sleep when they've been very physically active during the day. As adults, we can also reap the sleep benefits of daily exercise. In addition to daily aerobic exercise, like brisk dog walking, night time stretching can also help get us ready for sleep. Make an evening walk with Ginger and 15 minutes of gentle stretches after returning home part of your before-bed time routine.

- **CHANGE YOUR HOME ENVIRONMENT WITH NIGHT AND DAY CYCLES**

Before electricity, your brain could use changes in light conditions and sounds to help signal that it was time to go to sleep. When my boys went on camping trips with Scouts as kids, they'd always ask the leaders what time it was as dusk began to set. Since they did most of their camping during the school year, it could still be quite early when the skies were turning dark. The leaders would always answer, "Midnight!" and the boys would dash into their sleeping bags and soundly sleep until the sun rose to wake them. Even when we're old enough to read our own clocks, our brain will still respond to these same changes in our environment.

To help improve your sleep patterns, make it a habit to begin to dim the lights in your house and lower the volume of radios and televisions about one hour before your scheduled bed time. You may also wish to put a dim light on a timer to turn on about 30 to 60 minutes before you want to get up each morning, so your brain has time to prepare for waking up before the alarm blares.

- **HAVE A MILK AND CARBOHYDRATE SNACK IN THE EVENING**

Don't go to bed hungry. A calorie is a calorie—whether you eat it with breakfast or before bed. It's a myth that food eaten before bed turns into fat. So don't be afraid to add a small, healthy snack in the evening.

My dad always had a bowl of cereal before bed—taking advantage of the sleep-inducing benefits of milk and carbohydrates. Tryptophan and serotonin are important brain chemicals for sleep. Milk contains the protein tryptophan, which is why a glass of milk before bed can help with sleep. Warming the milk makes more tryptophan available to the brain. Other foods are also rich in these compounds. Part of the reason you feel so sleepy after Thanksgiving dinner is because turkey is also rich in tryptophan. So a glass of milk and turkey sandwich is a great evening snack when leftover turkey is around. Carbohydrates also change our levels of serotonin, making them a good bed time snack. So my dad's cold cereal and milk is often just what the doctor ordered for good sleep.

Adopt a regular sleep routine:

- Designate a spot for sleep
- Stick to regular bed and rising times
- Avoid caffeine and alcohol in the evening
- Exercise every day
- Do stretching exercises before gong to bed
- Dim the lights and lower noises
- Don't go to bed hungry

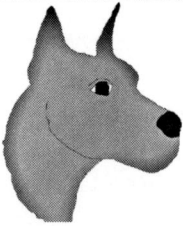

Chapter 5.

Be Man's Best Friend

> I always had plenty of friends in school and when I was working, but now that I've retired, I don't need friends like I used to. I get by fine with just my family and a couple neighbors I wave to. Fred C., Oil City, PA

People often refer to a dog as man's best friend. Dogs are great friends—they are loyal, trustworthy, and hold our secrets. A dog's friendship won't end because her human friend had a bad day, can't afford to take her out on the town, or wasn't attentive when struggling with a problem. George Eliot is quoted as having said, "Animals are such agreeable friends. They ask no questions. They pass no criticisms." (http://www.dog-names.org.uk/dog-quotes-quotations.htm. Accessed July 2008.) Studying our dogs can provide valuable insights into friendship and how to be a true friend.

You can begin to understand your dog's attitude toward his neighbors by comparing the behavior of humans and dogs when out for a stroll. Going for walks provides exercise and great opportunities for socializing. Humans and their dogs, however, approach walks with very different attitudes. Humans often feel nosy if they inspect the latest changes to their neighbor's garden or house. Humans will limit eye contact and conversation to close acquaintances only, sometimes even crossing the street to avoid encountering an unfamiliar neighbor. How often have you heard your own neighbors lament, "I've lived in this neighborhood for 15 years, and I still don't know who lives across the street from me!" When Duke goes for a walk, however, he's very focused on getting in touch with his community. As he sniffs the ground, mail box posts, and fire hydrants, he's gathering a wealth of information about his neighborhood dogs. "Fluffy must have switched dog food again." "Rascal down the street is really growing—he's marking much higher on the old scent post than the last time I sniffed it." "What's Butch doing leaving his scent near Bertie's mark? She's my bassett hound!" We humans often give our dogs a pathetic look, thinking, "You obviously don't have a care in the world when you can just waste time sniffing here and there." And if your dog sees another dog or human across the street—watch out! While you're trying to keep to a strict schedule with no interruptions, Lady will undoubtedly show her eagerness to cross the street to greet an old friend or make a new one. If you insist on ignoring a contact, you'll probably get "the look" from your dog that says, "Haven't you learned anything yet?! Being man's best friend is your most important work!" Buster has learned the benefits of being connected with his canine community. Take the quiz below to see if you know what benefits are in store for you when you take a lesson from Daisy and make man your best friend.

What benefits can you expect by being more involved in your community:
- ☐ Better mood
- ☐ Better eating habits
- ☐ Less heart disease
- ☐ Better long-term memory
- ☐ Longer life

Believe it or not, all of these can be important benefits of being more socially engaged. Numerous research studies have proven that taking an interest in your fellow man and being man's best friend significantly improve your outlook on life and your long-term health.

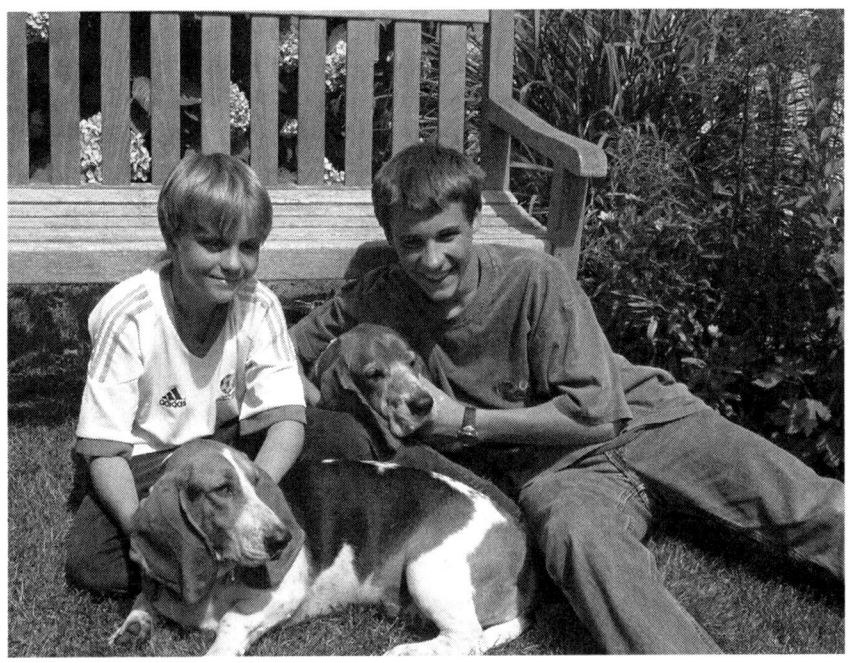

Learn to be a good companion from Phantom and Montgomery. (Photo courtesy of Julie Milone)

MAKE SOCIALIZING A PRIORITY

I really don't have time to worry about other people. I have enough to do to just take care of my own life. Roger H., Beaver Falls, PA

Have you ever watched a puppy move through a crowd of people? He'll stop to greet everyone. And not just for a minute—it's as though he wants to hear the details of everyone's life story. Before you rudely tug at his leash, stop and take a lesson from Rover. Taking a sincere interest in others around you isn't a waste of time, but an important way to improve your own health.

You might be surprised to learn that you can make your own life less stressful and more satisfying by getting involved with other people. Being socially engaged in your community and with family and friends will also improve your physical health. A lot of medical research has investigated the health impact from social involvement. A lack of friends is linked to poor health, while health improves for people who are socially involved (Zunzunegui 2004). Among older adults, general health continues to improve as the number of social activities increases (Zunzunegui 2004). Interestingly, older adults need more than simply involvement with family. In a large study of over 3000 seniors, being involved with networks of friends provided more health benefits than networks of only family and children (Zunzunegui 2004).

Researchers at Duke University reported their findings of social involvement and health in a large survey of almost 10,000 people (Barefoot 2005). In their study, more frequent interactions with family and friends resulted in about a 25 percent reduced risk for heart disease and death. It's pretty amazing that doing something as simple as checking in with friends, greeting your neighbors, and taking an interest in others can substantially improve your own well being and help you live a longer, healthier life.

YOU'RE NEVER TOO OLD TO NEED A FRIEND

It's been so hard to get my mother out of the house since dad died. She's just focused on her health and spends her day counting her pills and sleeping in front of the television.
Lisa Q., Weirton, WV

Growing old is tough work. It's easy to get discouraged and frustrated at our aging parents when they become less engaged. It's important to remember, however, that facing senior years takes great courage, fortitude, and perseverance. We adult children have to be respectful of the struggles our parents face and able to give them the space and freedom to make their own choices. Many older adults decrease their focus on other people, especially as close friends and siblings are lost. As their caring children, however, we must offer good opportunities for social engagement because of the many health benefits for seniors.

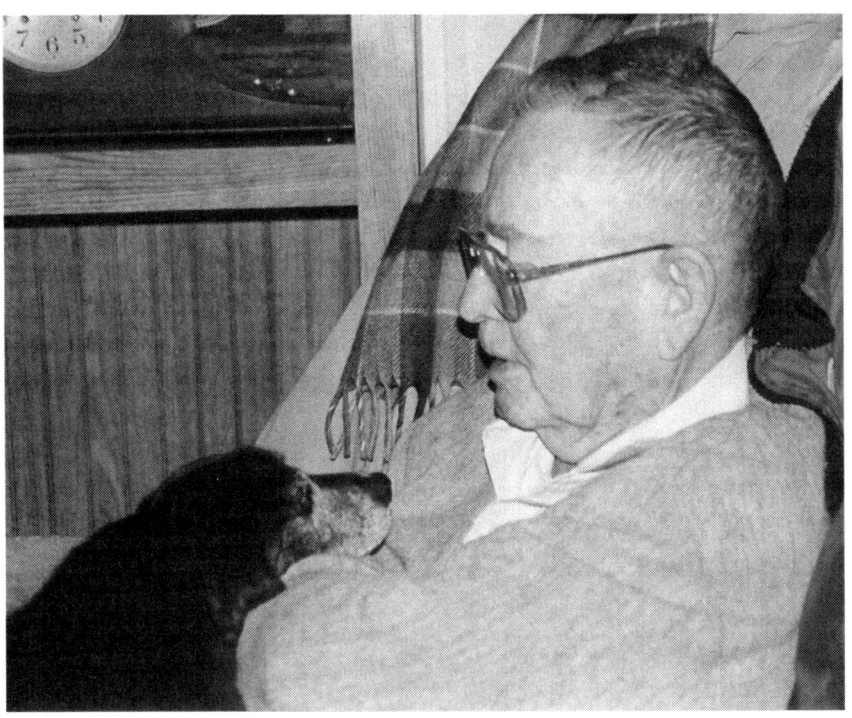

A couple of old friends sharing memories

Researchers in Australia followed senior citizens for 10 years (Giles 2005). In people 70 years old and older, the risk of dying decreased by 20 percent when people had a strong network of friends. Having social interactions with friends provided a greater effect than interactions with family members. So while we children may think that we and the grandkids should be enough to keep Grandpa engaged, it's essential that seniors develop relationships outside of their family. Visiting with and walking a quiet, well behaved dog can be a great way to help seniors shift focus from their own concerns onto those of other two- and four-legged friends.

Older people who are more socially engaged also develop fewer memory problems. Reduced involvement with relatives and friends has been linked to having worsened memory (Zunzunegui 2003). Fortunately, more social involvement has similarly been linked to a reduced rate of developing memory problems. In a study testing over 6000 seniors across about 5½ years, seniors having frequent social engagement had a slower decline in intellectual and memory abilities (Barnes 2004). Good mental capacity was maintained best in those people who were the most socially active. So chatting with neighbors and friends today may help keep the brain sharp for years to come.

Finally, eating is often an important social occasion and it's always more enjoyable to eat if you can share a meal. As people age, their diets often become more limited and many seniors lose an interest in eating. Having meals can become a chore rather than an occasion. Researchers at the University of Maryland proved that seniors with more social contacts ate better (Sahyoun 2005). Their diets were healthier, contained more nutritious calories, and included more fruits and vegetables compared with seniors with few social contacts. So whether you're able to eat with others or need to eat alone, having a strong network of friends and acquaintances results in healthier eating habits in the elderly.

Benefits for seniors from friendships and social engagement:

- Better general health
- Reduced risk for heart disease
- Improved memory
- Healthier eating habits

GET INVOLVED WITH YOUR COMMUNITY

I'm too busy with work and my kids to worry about making time for friends. Maybe I'll make friends a priority after my kids are in college.
Judy B., Scranton, PA

Before writing off the importance of friendships, let's ask Ginger about her thoughts on friendships. Most dogs love meeting other dogs and people. They're just as excited to greet a new contact as an old and dear friend. One of the hardest skills for my dog to learn in obedience classes was to be able to pass another dog without bounding over for a sniff and hello.

One of our early obedience lessons was to have Wheatie sit when he spotted a dog. He was trained to wait for the dog to approach, rather than tugging at the leash to get closer. Wheatie learned this lesson very well and during walks in populated areas will often stop abruptly and sit when he spies people or dogs in the distance. While I sometimes prefer to continue our walk and ignore the approaching folks, he seems to say, "Now this is important. Just sit quietly and wait a minute. It will be great to have a chance to say hello and hear their stories!" And I must admit, we've meet some of the nicest people while out on our walks who, without Wheatie, I would have scooted right by.

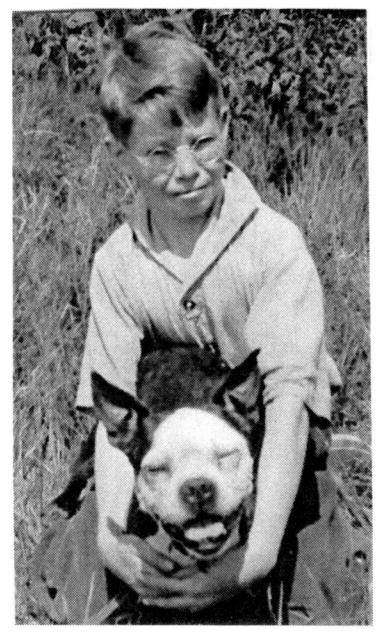

Friends enjoying each other's company

DON'T BE AFRAID TO BARK FOR ATTENTION

I've always been shy. It's really awkward trying to talk to other people. Ross P., Erie, PA

Use your dog as a conversation starter when acquaintances get together. It's always easier to start a conversation when there's something to use as an ice breaker other than the weather. When people walk with dogs, they often use their dogs to start conversations (Rogers 1993). Early discussions about your canine buddy can help turn a quick hello into a dialogue. Chatting about your dog's breed, what kind of obedience training you've done, and how long it takes to brush him every day, can easily extend into more personal conversations about work, family, and hobbies.

"This is Wheatie. He's just a year old. We got him at this time last year, during the AFC Championship game."

"Wasn't that a Cinderella series! I started to cry when Jerome won

the Super Bowl in his home town."
"What do you think Coach is going to do to help the season this year? It's been a disappointing season so far."
And before you know it, you've found that you're both huge Steelers fans and when you meet the next time on your walk, you'll probably talk about last week's game rather than just the nod or "hi" that might have passed for a conversation before your dog stopped to start a real conversation.

Having a dog to talk about can improve conversations in the neighborhood, pet-friendly stores, and even at businesses. Doctors in London found that more positive communications in the hospital occurred among family members, between patients, and between patients and their medical staff when a therapy dog was present (Cranz 1998). Just try to have a grouchy, complaining discussion with Buster staring you down with those big brown eyes, eagerly panting and wagging his tail. It's hard not to get a smile on your face and feel an instant improvement in attitude that you can easily share with others around you.

Still not convinced? Well, another benefit of keeping your dog with you as a conversation starter is that this will restrict visits to places where you might otherwise pick up unhealthy snacks. Sadly, most stores don't recognize the benefit of welcoming well-trained, leashed canines. Wheatie and I have found several welcoming stores in our area, which now get the bulk of our shopping business. Places where you might otherwise pop in for convenient, quick, sugar-filled snacks, however, typically will not permit your dog inside. It's much easier to pass by that cola, hot dog, and extra big chocolate bar on sale when you know Boxer can't go in; so you might as well keep walking and socializing, promoting much better long-term health.

Learn how to be a friend from Buster:

- Make social contacts a priority
- Don't miss opportunities to greet other people
- Take a genuine interest in others
- Use dog-talk as a conversation starter

PUT YOUR DOG TO WORK FOR YOU

My schedule is just too tight to try to fit in anything else. Patricia M., Titusville, PA

In today's over-structured world, we often look at time not dedicated to a specific task or down time as wasteful. If you're one of those people who just can't stand to have free time, put your dog to work and put Rover's work into your schedule. If you check with your local animal shelter, you'll probably find a number of programs designed to use your dog as a pet ambassador or therapy dog. As your dog's handler, you'll also need to attend these sessions and before you know it, you will have made a new network of dog-loving friends and become an eager volunteer!

Volunteering is a great way to get connected with other people and to start developing important relationships. According to statistics from the U.S. Department of Labor, about one in every 4 Americans volunteered through some organization during 2007. The average time spent volunteering during the year was 52 hours. When you volunteer, you can help a lot of other people. Medical research also shows that volunteering is great for *your* health. Both young and older people develop better health and an improved sense of life satisfaction when they volunteer (van Willigen 2000). As volunteer commitments increase, health benefits improve, up to a peak improvement when people are donating about 2 and ½ hours each week. People who volunteer more than that often find that volunteering becomes stressful and begins to interfere with their daily routine. Among seniors who volunteer, health benefits are greatest when they volunteer for more than one organization. Younger adults should concentrate their volunteer activities to a single organization. When younger adults volunteer with more than one group, their health benefits begin to diminish.

Many research studies have evaluated the health benefits of volunteering in senior citizens. Seniors often develop loneliness, depression, and worsening of physical health as they retire and have friends and close relatives die. Volunteering often helps fill an important gap for seniors. In addition, senior volunteers report better mood and health than those who don't volunteer (Morrow-Howell 2003). Formal volunteer programs can help provide an important new identify and purpose for older adults (Greenfield 2004). This new sense of purpose results in an improved life attitude, as well as the health benefits described above that go along with increasing social engagement.

Drs. Harris and Thoresen at Stanford University published their findings of a link between volunteering and mortality in the *Journal of Health Psychology* (Harris 2005). They monitored a sample of over 7500 seniors in the United States for 8 years. Compared to people who "never volunteered," people who "volunteered rarely" had a 41 percent decrease in mortality risk. People reporting they "sometimes volunteered" reduced their risk of death by 42 percent, while those "volunteering frequently" reduced their risk by 53 percent.

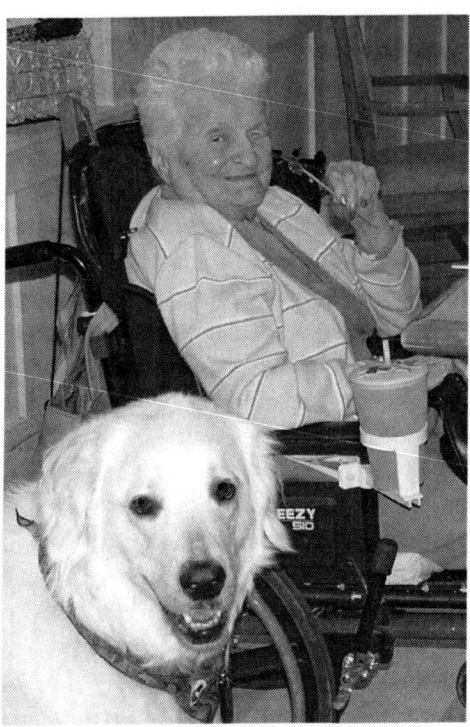

Let Bodhi help you start volunteering by becoming a therapy dog volunteer. (Photo courtesy of Joyce Arnowitz)

In most communities, there are numerous volunteer opportunities through religious organizations, hospitals, schools, etc. If you haven't volunteered for a while, let Duchess help you get started by doing volunteer work with your dog. When my dog was about 9 months old, we began taking a therapy dog class together to prepare for Canine Good Citizen and Therapy Dog International testing. Completing these tests shows that River is well mannered, interacts well with others, and reliably follows obedience commands. After completing our dog's certification, we humans also needed to complete an orientation. Our therapy instructor counseled, "Your dog will become your mentor and teach you what life is all about." Doing therapy visits with my dog has provided a great way to begin to share and care about other people. When visiting nursing homes, even residents who are reserved, disgruntled about their situation, or feeling under the weather can't help but brighten and get a smile when a friendly pooch walks in with eager eyes and a bright step. My son and I find that the residents look forward to their weekly visits from Wheatie and we look forward to checking in on our new "family" to see how they're faring each week.

Volunteering promotes positive community involvement:

- Volunteering helps provide a positive self-identity
- Volunteering is linked to better health
- Opportunities are available to volunteer with your dog
- Focus volunteer efforts with only one organization
- If you're retired, you might volunteer with two groups
- Limit volunteer time to about 2½ hours per week

Chapter 6.

Teach an Old Dog New Tricks

> I'm too old to learn new things. Computers, MP-3 players, email, and HD T.V. are all Greek to me. You can't teach an old dog new tricks, you know. Grace C., Hazelton, PA

Don't ever tell Flower that you can't teach an old dog new tricks. If you ask her, she'll probably insist that you *must* keep teaching your dog new tricks. Your dog will usually be eager to try out a new toy, a new walk, or even a new set of commands. Dogs understand the value of a life-long pattern of curiosity and an interest in new things. So teach an old "dog" new tricks by never missing an opportunity to learn and grow.

Researchers at the University of California surveyed 205 elderly people who were still living in the community about successful aging (Montross 2006). They defined successful aging as being able to live independently, readily adapt to changes, be engaged with others, be healthy, and have a strong sense of well-being and life satisfaction. Four factors were strongly linked to successful aging:

- Having more close friends
- Spending more days each week reading
- Spending more days each week listening to the radio
- Spending more days each week visiting family

This study shows that "staying connected" with the world, through reading, listening to the radio, and being engaged with friends and family, is what keeps us both mentally and physically strong as we age.

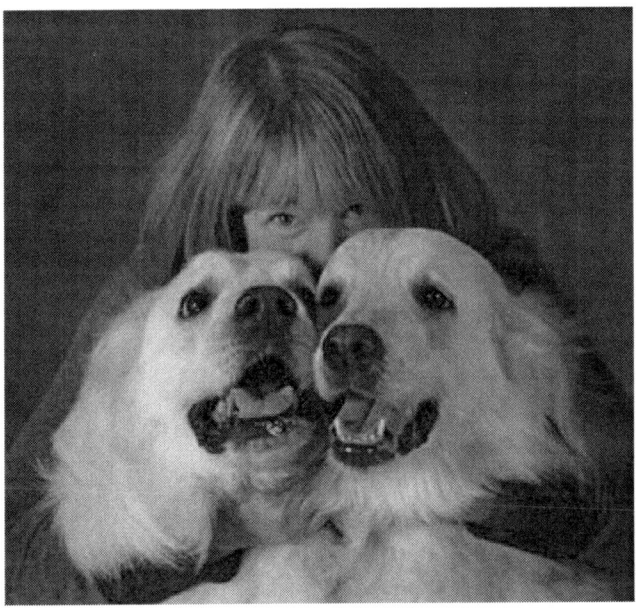

Be curious and keep investigating. (Photo courtesy of Joyce Arnowitz)

KEEP YOUR MIND ALERT

It's so hard to interest my parents in doing anything. They just plant themselves in front of the television for hours. I guess the T.V. keeps their minds busy. It's probably better than nothing. Jerry J., Tucson, AZ

As kids, we heard every day about how important it was to learn new things and keep our minds active and sharp. How often have we asked our own kids, "What did you learn at school today," expecting that every day will be a day to learn something new. Once we start our own families and careers, we sometimes forget to remind ourselves that learning is still important and exciting.

But what's the best way to keep our brains active and alert? Take this quiz to see if you can dig out those leisure activities that have been linked to good long-term mental health:
- ☐ Running
- ☐ Reading
- ☐ Watching television
- ☐ Weight training exercise
- ☐ Family board games

Your mind stays clearer in your senior years when you exercise your brain regularly. While mental activity does seem reduce your risk of developing memory problems, just doing physical exercise is less effective. Among those leisure activities listed above, reading and playing board games are the two that have been scientifically linked to better long-term mental abilities as we age.

The long-term benefits of keeping your mind alert were highlighted in a recent medical study. A group of almost 5500 adults over age 55 were followed for five years (Wang 2006). People who spent a lot of time watching television were much more likely to develop memory problems. Those people who would later develop memory problems reported watching television about twice as often as people whose memories stayed sharp. So when our moms told us that watching too much television was bad for us, they were probably right on the mark! Playing board games and reading, on the other hand, were linked to a reduced risk for developing memory problems. So keeping your mind alert today helps keep your brain sharp in the years to come.

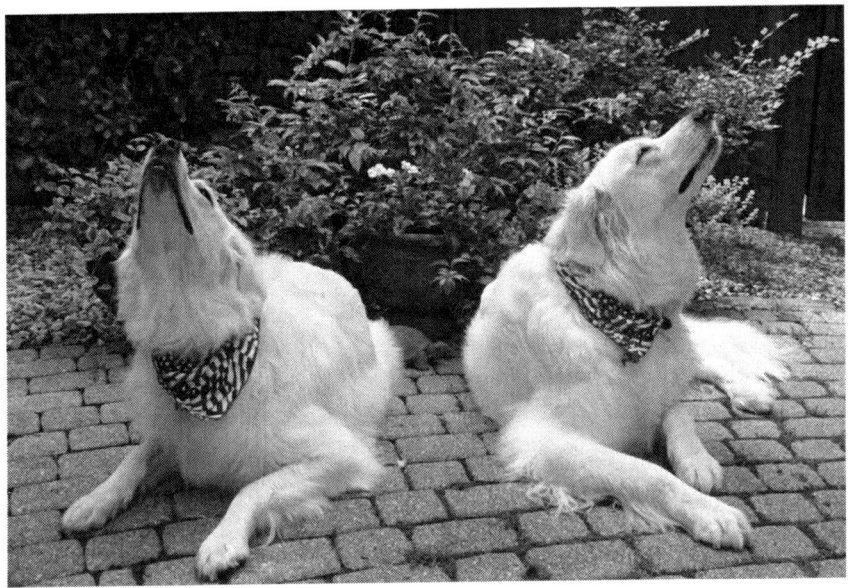

Take your cue from Bodhi and Sydney—sniff out new opportunities and adventures. (Photo courtesy of Joyce Arnowitz)

MAKE DUKE YOUR HOBBY WATCH DOG

I have a hard enough time getting my kids to do their homework and piano practice, let alone extra time to train a dog! Mary Lynne B., Washington, PA

Include Duke in your mental exercise and he might prove himself to be a great motivator for you. When I was a kid, I played the flute throughout middle school, high school, and college, although I always wanted to play the piano. We weren't able to afford a piano when I was growing up, but I nurtured that dream until I'd been in medical practice for a couple of years and could buy an electric keyboard. Through the years, my devotion to practice has waxed and waned and it's been very easy to get distracted by daily chores and then hard to get back to playing when feeling so far behind after missing so much practice time. As part of my dog's therapy dog training, he needed to learn a variety of commands. Dogs traditionally dislike the down command, because it puts them in a subordinate position, and my dog has always hated it. He would obediently lower his body near the ground, but not actually let his tummy touch the floor for a long time. To help work on down stays, I started having him sit by the piano when I practiced and do a long down stay until I finish practicing. I have a little dish of miniature doggie treats on the piano and every time I finish a song, he gets a little treat. Wheatens are not big barkers, but he barks once or twice if he has to go out or some other "urgent" request. If I miss my usual practice time, my dog now goes into the piano room, stands in his spot next to the bench and barks. When I come to see if he needs to go out, he just stands there and looks at the piano. Once I sit down, he lies down and goes to sleep. Who would have thought that I could train my dog to nag me into practicing my piano! Of course, I tell my friends and piano teacher that my dog is just very musical and loves to hear me play, but I suspect the treats are probably the attraction (although he now goes to sleep before getting a treat!). My piano teacher, aware of my level of skill, is, of course, skeptical that it's fine music the dog is seeking! It is self-reinforcing to have a demanding audience - "Look, Wheatie wants to hear me play!" It's too bad I didn't have this system in effect when I was badgering my two boys to stick to their piano lessons! Training your dog to sit for Junior's homework, spelling practice, or instrument practice can be a great way to help motivate your child to stick to his work, under the watchful and seemingly less nagging eye of Fluffy!

DIG INTO A GOOD BOOK

I really don't have time to read. I'd rather just relax in front of the television. Elsa W., Uniontown, PA

My oldest son wasn't interested in reading for pleasure until his fifth grade teacher added a series of *Hardy Boys* books to the classroom shelf. Like his mom, he devoured the mysteries and began what will hopefully be a life time of enthusiastic reading. For people who have gotten out of the habit of enjoying books, it's sometimes just a matter of finding something to spark your interest.

If you could take Pepper into the bookstore, he'd surely head for the dog book section. So follow his lead and include books about dogs and dog owners. Reading about your dog's breed or other people's experiences with their dogs can be a great way to keep yourself inspired to spend more healthy time with your own canine buddy.

Book stores and pet stores are stuffed with dog training books. My favorite is *Mother Knows Best*, by Carol Lea Benjamin. A professional dog trainer and author of several bestselling dog training books, Benjamin describes a training method that capitalizes on the natural instincts and expectations of your dog. She obviously loves dogs and helps the new owner take advantage of the natural desires of the dog that will make your pooch a welcome part of your family pack. Benjamin helps focus the owner on the canine motivations for "misbehavior," which usually stem from miscommunication about human expectations that would be foreign to a dog's natural instincts. Even though I'd grown up with dogs, I read it cover to cover and highlighted numerous passages to help train my new puppy when we got Wheatie. My dog-earred copy has proven to be a fabulous resource as well as a pleasure to read. Benjamin recently published a new training book, *See Spot Sit: 101 Illustrated Tips for Training the Dog You Love* that is sure to be a training standard. Patricia B. McConnell also has a number of useful training resources that target important training needs, such as *Beginning Family Dog Training* and *Puppy Primer*, which is co-authored with Brenda Scidmore. A good general dog information book is *Essential Dog. The Ultimate Guide to Owning a Happy and Healthy Pet* by Caroline Davis. And, of course, there are quite a number of popular dog training guides from television's *Dog Whisperer*, Cesar Millan.

I have a mature dog and we've already finished basic training, so I don't need to read anymore dog books. Leanne L., New Castle, PA

Hopefully Leader was out of earshot for this sentiment! There are a lot of other books available about dogs besides basic training guides. Reading books that highlight positive dog relationships will help strengthen your bond to Ranger.

My son developed his interest in mysteries from me. I grew up loving a good mystery and have devoured series by many authors. After having read a couple dozen *Cat Who* mysteries by Lillian Jackson Braun that feature Siamese cats, I was delighted to discover a series of mysteries focused on the dog world by poodle owner and author, Laurien Berenson. Her mysteries follow Melanie Travis, a young mom and poodle owner who stumbles upon and cleverly solves a variety of murder mysteries. Melanie breeds and shows standard poodles, and the reader will enjoy dog talk between Melanie and her dog friends inside and outside of the dog show circuit. Laurien Berenson's titles give you a hint of her great sense of humor, including *A Pedigree to Die For*, *Underdog*, *Dog Eat Dog*, *Hot Dog*, *Best in Show*, *Jingle Bell Bark*, *Chow Down*, and others. These mysteries are both entertaining and informative with lots of great tips about dog care and a glimpse into the sometimes glamorous world of show dogs.

Carol Lea Benjamin, author of my favorite dog training book (above), has also authored a series of detective stories focused on adult situations and themes, with a thoughtful social commentary included between murders and clues. Benjamin's main characters are detective Rachel Alexander and her pit bull partner, Dashiell. These stories give you a glimpse of the life of the working dog. Dashiell literally sniffs out clues as a detective assistant and also works as a therapy dog, visiting patients in nursing homes and AIDs facilities. In *Hell of a Dog*, Rachel and Dashiell ferret out a murderer while working undercover at a dog obedience seminar, allowing the reader to appreciate many different dog training techniques taught by Rachel's fellow instructors and suspects. Benjamin's books also include, *This Dog for Hire*, *The Dog Who Knew Too Much*, *The Long Good Boy*, *Without a Word*, and *The Hard Way*.

Several other mystery series that include dog owners and their canine companions, along with practical information about a variety of dog breeds and training techniques include:

- The Raine Stockton Dog Mysteries by Donna Ball
    - Dog trainer Raine Stockton solves mysteries in rugged and beautiful surroundings, like the Smoky Mountains.
    - Titles include: *Gun Shy*, *Smoky Mountain Tracks*, and *Rapid Fire*.
- The Holly Winter Mysteries by Susan Conant
    - Enjoy the adventures of dog writer, Holly Winter, and her two exuberant Alaskan malamutes.
    - Titles include: *Gaits of Heaven*, *Bride and Groom*, and *The Dogfather*.
- The Jack Field Mysteries by Lee Charles Kelley
    - Former detective and psychologist turned dog trainer, Jack Field, dishes out wise cracks and unconventional dog training while solving mysteries in Maine.

- Titles include: *Like a Dog with a Bone, Twas the Bite Before Christmas, Dogged Pursuit*
- *Bark M For Murder* is a collection of mysteries solved with the help of canine sleuths by J.A. Jance, Virginia Lanier, Chassie West, and Lee Charles Kelley, for those who would like a taste of several great writers.

Poetry lovers might enjoy reading the small collection of dog poems edited by Ferris Cook, *Bark: Selected Poems About Dogs*. These poems run the gamut from silly to serious by a variety of famous authors, including Robert Frost, Dorothy Parker, John Updike, and Ogden Nash. Another small collection of dog poems is *Doggerel: Poems About Dogs*, edited by Carmela Ciuraru.

If you prefer a novel, try Garth Stein's *The Art of Racing in the Rain*. In this novel, a wise lab-airedale mix walks the reader through the trials and turmoils facing a young man as he finds a bride, starts a family, becomes a widower, and finds a career driving race cars. Reading this book might get you thinking about how Rover interprets your behavior and reactions to daily strife.

If you prefer non-fiction books, several books have recently been published that highlight the benefits of a close relationship with your four-legged friend:

- *From Baghdad with Love* is a memoir of a Marine's experience in Iraq and how his military life was forever changed when he rescued an abandoned puppy during a military exercise.
- John O'Hurley, well known from his long-time role as J. Peterman on the *Seinfeld* comedy series, recently wrote a book describing his positive relationship with his dogs, *It's Okay to Miss the Bed on the First Jump and Other Life Lessons I Learned From Dogs*. This fun book is a quick read. Although there are not a lot of novel insights, the descriptions are fun and entertaining.
- Jack Canfield and colleagues have written another *Chicken Soup* book for animal lovers - *Chicken Soup for the Dog Lover's Soul*. As with other *Chicken Soup* books, you'd better have a box of tissues handy for this one!
- *Fitness Unleashed. A Dog Owner's Guide to Losing Weight and Gaining Health Together* by Marty Becker and Robert Kushner focuses on walking your dog to help drop pounds and become healthier.

- *The Dog Diet* by Patti Lawson is a memoir about how a divorced attorney's dysfunctional life became more structured and fulfilling once she introduced a shelter puppy into her home.
- *A Three Dog Life* by Abigail Thomas is the touching and courageous study of how a woman puts her life back together, with the help of her loving dogs, after her husband is disabled from a severe head injury.
- *Good Dog. Stay* by Anna Quindlen details how the author has grown through her relationship with her dog.

READ WITH ROVER

I'm sure reading would be good for me, but I just can't waste my day with pleasure reading. Rob W., New Kensington, PA

For those of you who just can't take time to smell the roses and enjoy the mental and physical benefits of relaxation, you can still experience the pleasure and gratification of reading by joining a dog reading program. Our local animal shelter sponsors a literacy program, called *Reading with Rover*. Similar programs are found in many areas. At our program, elementary school students who are struggling with reading are identified by their teachers for participation in the program. The child comes to a library to read to a certified therapy dog, who is accompanied by his handler. As the child reads, the dog listens intently and "corrects" the child when errors are made. Corrections are made by the handler saying things like, "Red didn't quite understand that sentence. Can you read it to him again?," or "Rusty doesn't know how to say that word either. Let me tell you both how it's pronounced," or "Cody really enjoyed that story. He liked the part where the dog found his boy again. He'd like to know what your favorite part was." Using the doggie dialogue, children are encouraged to accept corrections and read more "because Ginger would really like to hear another story." If your area doesn't offer these kinds of programs, be creative and work with your animal shelter volunteers to start a reading program for kids or shut-in seniors. Reading with the dog will be fun for you and those reading to the dog or listening to you read to them.

TAKE A CLASS

I used to enjoy drawing when I was younger, but I got tired of doing the same old landscape and still life scenes. Besides, I don't have the time or money to sign up for a class several days a week. Lucy T., Greenville, PA

If you think it might be fun to try something new or a novel twist on an old love, have a look at dog classes. Most large pet stores, kennels, and animal shelters offer a variety of dog classes. These can range from obedience, manners, agility, and rally classes for you and your dog to classes on dog care, dog photography, and even dog painting classes. Whatever your interest, you can probably find a class that will combine a long-lost hobby or pastime with your love of dogs. Taking a dog class can also provide you with the needed motivation to try something new.

Dog-focused classes are generally conveniently scheduled, economically priced, and of short duration so you don't usually need to make a big commitment. It's also easy to get to know other classmates, because you all have your dogs in common, providing an instant common bond. There's usually a lot of positive encouragement from both instructors and fellow classmates in most dog classes, with most classes focusing on strengthening the bond between you and your dog and your dog's ability to positively interact with other people and dogs.

Stay mentally active throughout life:

- Keep your mind alert
- Dig into a good book
- Join a class
- Volunteer in a literacy or reading program

Chapter 7.

Live a Dog's Life

So now you have the facts—living the dog's life will keep you healthier, happier, and more mentally alert and you'll even live longer. As you can see from the earlier chapters, there is more than just a handful of research studies suggesting that having a dog in your life and as your guide will improve your health. An abundance of studies have been conducted at some of the finest medical centers across in the world, testing large groups of people for long periods of time. The verdict is definitely in—Rover is GREAT for your physical and mental health!

This chapter will give you some last minute tips about how to put everything you've learned together to start effectively living "a dog's healthy life."

MAKE YOURSELF A SCHEDULE

Before Wheatie came home, we posted a puppy training schedule on the refrigerator, listing times for potty breaks, walks, kennel time, meals, etc. We stuck to the schedule religiously for the first couple of months and his behavior was great and housebreaking accidents infrequent. Laziness resulted in straying from the schedule, with resultant behavior problems and "surprises" left in the dining room. We soon learned that, like my boys, Wheatie did best with a consistent schedule in place.

So make a schedule for yourself—include daily times for four essential daily activities:

- Sleeping
- Meals
- Exercise
- Socializing

Make your schedule specific—listing when, where, and how you plan to sleep, eat, exercise, and socialize. You can use the sample daily *Fit As Fido* living a dog's life log provided in this chapter. (See Chart 1.) Read the completed sample schedule (Chart 2) to give you ideas about how to individualize your own calendar.

Sample daily *Fit As Fido* living a dog's life log

	When	Where	How
Waking up			
Breakfast			
Lunch			
Dinner			
Snacks			
Exercise			
Socializing			
Bed time			

Chart 1 instructions: Complete this log for your typical week day. Include specific details about the time of day when each task should be scheduled (when) and the place where you will do each task (where). In the how column, give yourself suggestions about how to best accomplish the task—what strategies you will use to help achieve your target goal.

Sample completed daily *Fit As Fido* living a dog's life log

	When	Where	How
Waking up	6:30 a.m.	Bed	Set lights to begin to turn on in bedroom starting at 6 a.m. Set percolator to start making coffee at 7 a.m.
Breakfast	7:15 a.m.	Kitchen	Eat a quiet breakfast while reading the newspaper
Lunch	11:30 a.m.	Work cafeteria	Eat with coworkers rather than while answering calls at my desk
Dinner	7:00 p.m.	Dining room	Make family meal time a special event each night
Snacks	5:15 p.m.	At home before going to the park	Water bottle and fresh fruit
Exercise	7 a.m.—10 minute walk with Chelsea before work. 5:30 p.m.—20 minute walk with Chelsea in the park before preparing dinner. 9:30 p.m.—10 minute walk with Chelsea before bed.	Do morning and late evening walks in the neighborhood. Go to the off-leash park for a longer walk after work.	Do the morning walk before the kids get up to get ready for school. Keep leash and other dog supplies in the car so I can quickly pick up Chelsea after work for the park. Plan the evening walk for after the kids are tucked in bed and asleep.

Socializing	Lunch During time at the park Family dinner	Have lunch at the cafeteria with the girls. Dog walking with Chelsea in the park. Dinner in the kitchen.	Eat lunch with co-workers. Chat with other dog owners at the park after work and before dinner. Plan to have the whole family eat dinner together after the kids come home from practice.
Bed time	10:30 p.m.	Go to bed only when it's time to go to sleep	Turn lights down around 9:30 p.m. and do 15 minutes of relaxation techniques and stretches before bed.

Remember—you should set the following targets for yourself:
- Meals
  - Make time to sit down for a meal—preferably with others
  - Plan to consume your calories during meal time and not in between meals
  - If you need a snack, have a large glass of water plus fresh fruit or crunchy vegetables
- Exercise
  - Plan to exercise a total of 150 minutes of moderate intensity, aerobic exercise (like brisk walking or hiking with Finnegan) each week
  - Try to exercise about 30 minutes per day, at least five days per week
  - Don't try to do all of your exercise in one long session
  - Vary your exercise so you don't get bored
  - Keep yourself well hydrated
- Sleep
  - 10 hours nightly if you're a pre-teen child
  - 9 hours per night if you're a teenager
  - 7-8 hours per night if you're an adult

- Consider including one 30-minute, mid-afternoon nap each day
• Socialize
  - Plan encounters with family, friends, and strangers
  - Take advantage of unexpected opportunities to connect with others in your community
  - Use Boo as an icebreaker
  - Take advantage of socializing opportunities during scheduled meals and exercise to interact with others

After making a schedule—chart your progress. You can use the walking log in Chapter 3 to monitor your exercise program. You can also chart your eating, sleeping, exercising, and socializing, using the sample weekly *Fit As Fido* progress chart provided below (Chart 3). Keeping tabs on your behavior will motivate you to follow Rocky's lessons, encourage you when you see positive improvements in your behavior, and help you catch lapses in good behavior when they first start to occur.

Sample weekly *Fit As Fido* progress chart

	Sun	Mon	Tues	Wed	Thurs	Fri	Sat
Eating							
3 meals							
Good portions							
Healthy choices							
Sleeping							
7-8 hours at night							
Exercising							
30 minutes, moderate intensity aerobic exercise							
Socializing							
Spent time with others							

Chart 3 instructions: Chart your progress every day by checking the appropriate boxes if you successfully achieve your target task. Remember—you don't have to be perfect every day for success. Review your charts to make sure you do a little better job of living the dog's life of good health each week.

REMEMBER THAT FOOD IS FOR NUTRITION

Bailey knows that food's for nourishment—not emotional comfort or a substitute for physical or mental stimulation. Fill your diet with the same kinds of good, healthy nutrients you see pictured on Charlie's dog food bag:

- Protein
    - Have nuts each day, including healthy almonds, walnuts, and nut butters
- Whole grains
    - Choose cereals rich in healthy oats
    - Select whole grain instead of white breads
- Fruits
    - Have fruits at each meal
    - Keep a bowl of washed fruit in the refrigerator and on the counter to help you choose a whole fruit as a snack. Remember—an apple a day IS a healthy way to consume healthy nutrients.
    - Include healthy citrus fruits (including tomatoes), blueberries, and cranberries in your diet
- Vegetables
    - Have vegetables at most meals
    - Keep washed and cut vegetables in the refrigerator for quick, healthy snacks (celery and carrot sticks, radishes, cucumber slices, etc.)
    - Eat fresh salads with dark, green, leafy vegetables
    - Add onions and garlic to your recipes

Keep yourself hydrated by drinking at least 8-10 cups of water each day, with more added when you exercise. Make sure you drink before and after each exercise session. Keep water available for you and Barney during exercise.

RELIEVE BOREDOM, THE BLUES, ANXIETY, AND STRESS WITH ACTIVITY

The first thing to do when you feel bored or distressed is to get up and get moving. Exercising where you will likely run into others for socialization is ideal. So grab Harley and his leash and head outside. If the weather truly prevents you from getting out, head for the nearest pet store and enjoy an afternoon of browsing through the aisles with Harley. Make sure you chat with others in the store—say hello to the customer with the poodle, ask the man with the giant bag of dog food what kind of dog he has at home, ask the sales clerk to compare a couple dog products for you.

MENTALLY CHALLENGE YOURSELF THROUGHOUT YOUR LIFE

Every adult should be learning and challenging him or herself. Look for opportunities to challenge yourself to learn something new—don't worry that you'll be the oldest person, the only female, or the least skilled student in the class. You can find classes at community centers, local colleges, and some stores. Maggie might suggest classes through your local pet stores or animal shelter.

Use quiet time to keep your brain engaged. Curl up with a good book and Coco for a relaxing evening. Or call the family or friends together and pull out board games. Remember—reading and playing board games are important mentally-stimulating activities that keep your brain alert as you age.

When in doubt—put on your walking shoes, grab the leash and a water bottle, whistle for Lucy, and go out for a walk or to the park. Walking will give you both physical and mental stimulation, provide opportunities for socializing with others out doing the same thing, and prevent you from falling back into bad habits. If you're still not convinced, ask Daisy, "You want to go for a walk?" Her big smile and wagging tail will let you know the answer is a definite yes!

Try volunteering. Remember that volunteering should be fun and not drudgery. Limit your volunteering as follows:

- Only volunteer for one organization
  - You can volunteer for two organizations if you're retired
- Maximum of 2½ hours weekly

Once people know you are an eager volunteer, you'll likely find too many volunteer opportunities are offered to you. Don't be tempted to volunteer for too much or for every activity your children might get involved in. You'll be a more productive volunteer and better parent at home if you set boundaries for your volunteer commitments.

DON'T KEEP YOURSELF IN THE DOG HOUSE

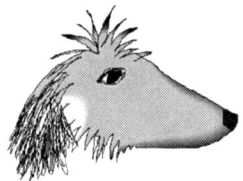

Remember—no one's perfect. Even Princess will have bad days when she sneaks scraps off the table, chews a table leg, or has an accident in the house. Expect that you'll also land in the dog house now and then by eating too much, sleeping too little, watching television instead of walking Sandy, or isolating yourself. When this happens, like Abby, lick your wounds for a few minutes, then get out of the dog house and back on the path to better health. Following a dog's life is hard work—maybe that's why Dakota sleeps so much! Expects some bumps along the way and most importantly remember—your health will improve even with small, consistent changes in your lifestyle habits. The more improvements you make—the better your health. But every little bit helps. So if you're having a bad day or bad week—don't despair—don't give up—don't just sit in the dog house. Get up—get the leash—get outside—get moving—get engaged with your community—and get healthy. Live the dog's life!

References

Allen K, Blascovich J, Mendes WB. Cardiovascular reactivity and the presence of pets, friends, and spouses: the truth about cats and dogs. *Psychosomatic Med* 2002;64:727-739.

Anderson WP, Reid CM, Jennings GL. Pet ownership and risk factors for cardiovascular disease. *Med J Aust* 1992;157:298-301.

Andres-Lacueva C, Shukitt-Hale B, Galli RL, et al. Anthocyanins in aged blueberry-fed rats are found centrally and may enhance memory. *Nutr Neurosci* 2005;8:111-120.

Ayas NT, White DP, Manson JE, et al. A prospective study of sleep duration and coronary heart disease in women. *Arch Intern Med* 2003;163:205-209.

Barefoot JC, Gronbaek M, Jensen G, Schnohr P, Prescott E. Social network diversity and risks of ischemic heart disease and total mortality: findings from the Copenhagen City Heart Study. *Am J Epidemiol* 2005;161:960-967.

Barnes LL, Mendes de Leon CF, Wilson RS, Bienias JL, Evans DA. Social resources and cognitive decline in a population of older African Americans and whites. *Neurology* 2004;63:2322-2326.

Basu A, Imrhan V. Tomatoes versus lycopene in oxidative stress and carcinogenesis: conclusions from clinical trials. *Eur J Clin Nutr* 2007;61:295-303.

Bauman AE, Russell SJ, Furber SE, Dobson AJ. The epidemiology of dog walking: an unmet need for human and canine health. *Med J Aust* 2001;175:632-634.

Blackman MR. Age-related alterations in sleep quality and neuroendocrine function. Interrelationships and implications. *JAMA* 2000;284:879-881.

Boyer J, Liu RH. Apple phytochemicals and their health benefits. *Nutr J* 2004;3:5.

Brown WJ, Ford JH, Burton NW, Marshall AL, Dobson AJ. Prospective study of physical activity and depressive symptoms in middle-aged women. *Am J Prev Med* 2005;29:265-272.

Brown SG, Rhodes RE. Relationships among dog ownership and leisure-time walking in western Canadian adults. *Am J Prev Med* 2006;30:131-136.

Bryant PA, Trinder J, Curtis N. Sick and tired: does sleep have a vital role in the immune system? *Nat Rev* 2004;4:457-467.

Burger KS, Kern M, Coleman KJ. Characteristics of self-selected portion size in young adults. *J Am Diet Assoc* 2007;107:611-618.

Cajochen C, Münch M, Knoblauch V, Blatter K, Wirz-Justice A. Age-related changes in the circadian and homeostatic regulation of human sleep. Chronobiol Int 2006;23:461-474.

CDC (Centers for Disease Control and Prevention). State-specific prevalence of obesity among adults—United States, 2005. *Morb Mortal Wkly Rep* 2006;55:985-988.

Chambliss HO. Exercise duration and intensity in a weight-loss program. *Clin J Sport Med* 2005;15:113-115.

Chubak J, McTiernan A, Sorensen B, et al. Moderate-intensity exercise reduces the incidence of colds among postmenopausal women. *Am J Med* 2006;119:937-942.

Claustrat B, Loisy C, Brun J, et al. Nocturnal plasma melatonin levels in migraine: a preliminary report. *Headache* 1989;29:242-245.

Colliard L, Ancel J, Benet J, Paragon B, Blanchard G. Risk factors for obesity in dogs in France. *J Nutr* 2006;136:1951S-1954S.

Cranz D. Animal-assisted therapy: assessing the benefits. *J Small Anim Pract* 1998;39:310-311.

Das S, Otani H, Maulik N, Das DK. Lycopene, tomatoes, and coronary heart disease. *Free Radic Res* 2005;39:449-455.

Dembicki D, Anderson J. Pet ownership may be a factor in improved health of the elderly. *J Nutr Elder* 1996;15:15-31.

Dhand R, Sohal H. Good sleep, bad sleep! The role of daytime naps in healthy adults. *Curr Opin Pulm Med* 2006;12:379-382.

Duthie SJ, Jenkinson AM, Crozier A, et al. The effects of cranberry juice consumption on antioxidant status and biomarkers relating to heart disease and cancer in healthy human volunteers. *Eur J Nutr* 2006;45:113-122.

Friedmann E, Thomas SA. Pet ownership, social support, and one-year survival after acute myocardial infarction in the Cardiac Arrhythmia Suppression Trial (CAST). *Am J Cardiol* 1995;76:1213-1217.

Galeone C, Pelucchi C, Levi F, et al. Onion and garlic use and human cancer. *Am J Clin Nutr* 2006;84:1027-1032.

Galper DI, Trivedi MH, Barlow CE, Dunn AL, Kampert JB. Inverse association between physical inactivity and mental health in men and women. *Med Sci Sports Exerc* 2006;38:173-178.

Gangwisch JE, Heymsfield SB, Boden-Albala B, et al. Short sleep duration as a risk factor for hypertension. Analyses of the first

National Health and Nutrition Examination Survey. *Hypertension* 2006;47:833-839.

Gangwisch JE, Malaspina D, Boden-Albala B, Heymsfield SB. Inadequate sleep as a risk factor for obesity: analyses of the NHANES I. *Sleep* 2005;28:1289-1296.

Giles LC, Glonek GV, Luszcz MA, Andrews GR. Effect of social networks on 10 year survival in very old Australians: the Australian longitudinal study of aging. *J Epidemiol Community Health* 2005;59:574-579.

Gottselig JM, Adam M, Retey JV, et al. Random number generation during sleep deprivation: effects of caffeine on response maintenance and stereotypy. *J Sleep Res* 2006;15:31-40.

Greenfield EA, Marks NF. Formal volunteering as a protective factor for older adults' psychological well-being. *J Gerontol* 2004;59B:S258-S264.

Ham SA, Epping J. Dog walking and physical activity in the United States. *Prev Chronic Dis* 2006;3:A47.

Harris AH, Thoresen CE. Volunteering is associated with delayed mortality in older people: analysis of the longitudinal study of aging. *J Health Psychol* 2005;10:739-752.

Hayashi M, Motoyoshi N, Hori T. Recuperative power of a short daytime nap with or without stage 2 sleep. *Sleep* 2005;28:829-836.

Howarth NC, Huang TK, Roberts SB, Lin B, McCrory MA. Eating patterns and dietary composition in relation to BMI in younger and older adults. *Int J Obes* 2007;31:675-684.

Irwin MR, Wang M, Campomayor CO, Collado-Hidalgo A, Cole S. Sleep deprivation and activation of morning levels of cellular and genomic markers of inflammation. *Arch Intern Med* 2006;166:1756-1762.

Jakicic JM, Wing RR, Butler BA, Robertson RJ. Prescribing exercise in multiple short bouts versus one continuous bout: effects on adherence, cardiorespiratory fitness, and weight loss in overweight women. *Int J Obes Relat Metab Disord* 1995;19:893-901.

Jambazian PR, Haddad E, Rajaram S, Tanzman J, Sabaté J. Almonds in the diet simultaneously improve plasma α-tocopheral concentrations and reduce plasma lipids. *J Am Diet Assoc* 2005;105:449-454.

Jiang R, Manson JE, Stampfer MJ, Liu S, Willett WC, Hu FB. Nut and peanut butter consumption and risk of type 2 diabetes in women. *JAMA* 2002;228:2554-2560.

Kavouras SA. Assessing hydration status. *Curr Opin Clin Nutr Metab Care* 2002;5:519-524.

Kelly JH, Sabate J. Nuts and coronary heart disease: an epidemiological perspective. *Br J Nutr* 2006;96(suppl 2):S61-S67.

Kelman L, Rains JC. Headache and sleep: examination of sleep patterns and complaints in a large clinical sample of migraineurs. *Headache* 2005;45:904-910.

Kienzle E, Bergler R, Mandernach. A comparison of the feeding behavior and the human-animal relationship in owners of normal and obese dogs. *J Nutr* 1998;128:2779S-2782S.

Knutson KL, Ryden AM, Mander BA, van Cauter E. Role of sleep duration and quality in the risk and severity of Type 2 diabetes mellitus. *Arch Intern Med* 2006;166:1768-1774.

Kotake-Nara E, Kushiro M, Zhang H, et al. Carotenoids affect proliferation of human prostate cancer cells. *J Nutr* 2001;131:3303-3306.

Kruger J, Galuska DA, Serdula MK, Jones DA. Attempting to lose weight. Specific practices among U.S. adults. *Am J Prev Med* 2004;26:402-406.

Kruk J. Physical activity in the prevention of the most frequent chronic diseases: an analysis of the recent evidence. *Asian Pac J Cancer Prev* 2007;8:325-338.

Lang T, Dimitriov S, Fehm H, Westermann J, Born J. Shift of monocyte function toward cellular immunity during sleep. *Arch Intern Med* 2006;116:1695-1700.

Lee I, Skerrett PJ. Physical activity and all-cause mortality: what is the dose-response relation? *Med Sci Sports Exerc* 2001;33(6 Suppl):S459-S71.

Ma Y, Bertone ER, Stanek EJ, et al. Association between eating patterns and obesity in a free-living US adult population. *Am J Epidemiol* 2003;158:85-92.

Macera CA, Ham SA, Yore MM, et al. Prevalence of physical activity in the United States: behavioral risk factor surveillance system, 2001. *Prev Chronic Dis* 2005;2:A17.

Mallon L, Broman J, Hetta J. High incidence of diabetes in men with sleep complaints or short sleep duration. *Diabetes Care* 2005;28:2762-2767.

Manz F, Wentz A. The importance of good hydration for the prevention of chronic diseases. *Nutr Rev* 2005;63:S2-S5.

Marsh AP, Katula JA, Pacchia CF, et al. Effect of treadmill and overground walking on function and attitudes in older adults. *Med Sci Sports Exerc* 2006;38:1157-1164.

Matsubara K, Matsumoto H, Mizushina Y, et al. Inhibitory effect of glycolipids from spinach on in vitro and ex vivo angiogenesis. *Oncol Rep* 2005;14:157-160.

McGreevy PD, Thomson PC, Pride C, et al. Prevalence of obesity in dogs examined by Australian veterinary practices and the risk factors involved. *Vet Rec* 2005;156:695-702.

McNicholas J, Collis GM. Dogs as catalysts for social interactions: robustness of the effect. *Br J Psychol* 2000;91:61-70.

Montross LP, Depp C, Daly J, et al. Correlates of self-rated successful aging among community-dwelling older adults. *Am J Geriatr Psychiatry* 2006;14:43-51.

Morris MC, Evans DA, Tangney CC, Bienias JL, Wilson RS. Associations of vegetable and fruit consumption with age-related cognitive change. *Neurology* 2006;67:1370-1376.

Morrow-Howell N, Hinterlong J, Rozario PA, Tang F. Effects of volunteering on the well-being of older adults. *J Gerontol* 2003;58B:S137-S145.

Murtagh EM, Boreham CA, Nevill A, Hare LG, Murphy MH. The effects of 60 minutes of brisk walking per week, accumulated in two different patterns, on cardiovascular risk. *Prev Med* 2005;41:92-97.

Myers J, Kaykha A, George S, et al. Fitness versus physical activity patterns in predicting mortality in men. *Am J Med* 2004;117:912-918.

Nakamura Y, Tanaka K, Yabushita N, Sakai T, Shigematsu R. Effects of exercise frequency on functional fitness in older adult women. *Arch Gerontol Geriatr* 2007;44:163-73.

Naska A, Oikonomou E, Trichopoulou A, et al. Siesta in healthy adults and coronary mortality in the general population. *Arch Intern Med* 2007;167:296-301.

National Sleep Foundation 2008 Sleep in America Poll. Available at www.sleepfoundation.org. Accessed July 2008.

Nielsen SJ, Popkin BM. Patterns and trends in food portions sizes, 1997-1998. *JAMA* 2003;289:450-453.

Nies MA, Motyka CL. Factors contributing to women's ability to maintain a walking program. *J Holistic Nursing* 2006;24:7-14.

Noyes R, Carney CP, Hillis SL, Jones LE, Langbehn DR. Prevalence and correlates of illness worry in the general population. *Psychosomatics* 2005;46:529-539.

O'Dowd A. More than 12 million adults in England will be obese by 2010. *BMJ* 2006;333:463.

Ohayon MM. Prevalence and correlates of nonrestorative sleep complaints. *Arch Intern Med* 2005;165:35-41.

Pearson NJ, Johnson LL, Nahin RL. Insomnia, trouble sleeping, and complementary and alternative medicine. Analysis of the 2002 National Health Interview Survey. *Arch Intern Med* 2006;166:1775-1782.

Rai A, Mohapatra SC, Shukla HS. Correlates between vegetable consumption and gallbladder cancer. *Eur J Cancer Prev* 2006;15:134-137.

Raina P, Waltner-Toews D, Bonnett B, Woodard C, Abernathy T. Influence of companion animals on the physical and psychological health of older people: an analysis of a one-year longitudinal study. *J Am Geriatr Soc* 1999;47:323-329.

Ritz R, Berrut G. The importance of good hydration for day-to-day health. *Nutr Rev* 2005;63:S6-S13.

Roehrs T, Hyde M, Blaisdell B, Greenwald M, Roth T. Sleep loss and REM sleep loss are hyperalgesic. *Sleep* 2006;29:145-151.

Rogers J, Hart LA, Boltz RP. The role of pet dogs in casual conversations of elderly adults. *J Soc Psychol* 1993;133:265-277.

Romero AL, Romero JE, Galaviz S, Fernandez ML. Cookies enriched with psyllium or oat bran lower plasma LDL cholesterol in normal and hypercholesterolemic men from Northern Mexico. *J Am Coll Nutr* 1998;17:601-608.

Sahyoun NR, Zhang XL. Dietary quality and social contact among a nationally representative sample of the older adult population in the United States. *J Nutr Health Aging* 2005;9:177-183.

Serpell J. Beneficial effects of pet ownership on some aspects of human health and behaviour. *J Royal Soc Med* 1991;84:717-720.

Siegel JM. Stressful life events and use of physician services among the elderly: the moderating role of pet ownership. *J Pers Soc Psychol* 1990;58:1081-1086.

Spiegel K, Knutson K, Leproult R, Tasali E, Van Cauter E. Sleep loss: a novel risk factor for insulin resistance and Type 2 diabetes. *J Appl Physiol* 2005;99:2008-2019.

Steptoe A, Peacey V, Wardle J. Sleep duration and health in young adults. *Arch Intern Med* 2006;166:1689-1692.

Takase B, Akima T, Satomura K, et al. Effects of chronic sleep deprivation on autonomic activity by examining heart rate variability, plasma catecholamine, and intracellular magnesium levels. *Biomed Pharmacother* 2004;58 (suppl 1):S35-S39.

Vanitallie TB. Sleep and energy balance: interactive homeostatic systems. *Metabolism* 2006;55 (10 suppl 2):S30-S35.

Van Willigen M. Differential benefits of volunteering across the life course. *J Gerontol* 2000;55B:S308-S318.

Voelker R. Studies suggest dog walking a good strategy for fostering fitness. *JAMA* 2006;296:643.

Wang JJ, Zhou DD, Li J, et al. Leisure activity and risk of cognitive impairment: the Chongquip aging study. *Neurology* 2006;66:911-913.

Wang Y, Chang CF, Chou J, et al. Dietary supplementation with blueberries, spinach, or spirulina reduces ischemic brain damage. *Exp Neurol* 2005;193:75-84.

Warburton DR, Nicol CW, Bredin AD. Prescribing exercise as preventive therapy. *CMAJ* 2006;174:961-974.

Wilson CC. The pet as an anxioloytic intervention. *J Nerv Ment Dis* 1991;179:482-489.

Wilson MA, Shukitt-Hale B, Kalt W, et al. Blueberry polyphenols increase lifespan and thermotolerance in *Caenorhabditis elegans*. *Aging Cell* 2006;5:59-68.

Wu Y. Overweight and obesity in China. *BMJ* 2006;333:362-363.

Yaggi HK, Araujo AB, McKinlay JB. Sleep duration as a risk factor for the development of Type 2 diabetes. *Diabetes Care* 2006;29:657-661.

Young LR, Nestle M. Portion sizes and obesity: responses of fast-food companies. *J Public Health Policy* 2007;28:238-248.

Zhang L, Samet J, Caffo B, Punjabi NM. Cigarette smoking and nocturnal sleep architecture. *Am J Epidemiol* 2006;164:529-537.

Zunzunegui M, Alvardo BE, Del Ser T, Otero A. Social networks, social integration, and social engagement determine cognitive decline in community-dwelling Spanish older adults. *J Gerontol* 2003;58B:S93-S100.

Zunzunegui M, Koné A, Johri M, et al. Social networks and self-rated health in two French-speaking Canadian community dwelling populations over 65. *Soc Sci Med* 2004;58:2069-2081.

Breinigsville, PA USA
17 August 2010
243687BV00002B/21/P